Dr Valerie Hey is a researcher based at the Social Science Research Unit, Institute of Education, University of London. She is writing a book about girls' friendship drawing upon her own research, provisionally titled *The Company She Keeps: Ethnographies of girls' friendships*. She lives in London with her two daughters, Laura Grace and Esther Kate.

Dr Catherine Itzin is Research Professor in Social Care and Public Policy in the School of Social and International Studies at the University of Sunderland. She is the editor and co-author of *Pornography: Women, Violence and Civil Liberties* (1992) and *Gender, Culture and Organisational Change* (1995).

Lesley Saunders is a researcher in education. She is a published poet and performs with the Bloody Poets; she won the George MacBeth Award in 1993, and the *Guardian* Women's Poetry competition in 1994; and edited *Glancing Fires: An Investigation into Women's Creativity* (The Women's Press, 1987).

Mary Anne Speakman lectured in sociology and women's studies at the Open University, before engaging in freelance writing and research. She now teaches child studies to nursery nursing students, and lives in Cardiff with Terry Marsden and their children, Hannah and Joseph.

GW00648547

Also edited by Lesley Saunders from The Women's Press:

Glancing Fires: An Investigation into Women's Creativity (1987)

**VALERIE HEY, CATHERINE ITZIN,
LESLEY SAUNDERS &
MARY ANNE SPEAKMAN,
EDITORS**

Hidden
Loss

Miscarriage & Ectopic
Pregnancy

**SECOND EDITION
FULLY REVISED AND UPDATED**

**THIS EDITION EDITED
BY KATE MOSSE**

First published by The Women's Press Ltd, 1989
A member of the Namara Group
34 Great Sutton Street, London EC1V 0DX

Reprinted and revised 1996

Grateful acknowledgment is made for permission to reprint the lines
from the poem 'The Moon is Always Female' from *The Moon is
Always Female* by Marge Piercy, Alfred A Knopf, Inc, 1981, © Marge
Piercy.

Figure 4 is based on a diagram in *The Cervical Stitch: What It's Like*
by Ros Kane.

British Library Cataloguing-in-Publication Data
Hidden Loss
    1. Women. Miscarriages. Personal Adjustment
    I. Hey, Valerie
    306.8'8

ISBN 0 7043 4457 2

Typeset in Times Roman by Contour Typesetters, Southall, London
Printed and bound in Great Britain by BPC Paperbacks Ltd

To the unborn ones

Out of necessity's hard stones we suck
what water we can and so we have survived,
women born of women.

Marge Piercy
'The Moon is Always Female'

Contents

Part Five:
Appendices

Figures

Acknowledgments

Many people helped in the production of the first edition of this book, whether by telling us their stories, giving timely advice or offering practical and emotional support. In particular, we wanted to thank wholeheartedly those women who shared with us their experiences, especially those who relived the pain by writing up their accounts for the book; their courage continues to shine through ten years later. We were also grateful to Sheila White for the illustrations and to Catherine Henderson for her guidance on alternative medicine. We wanted to express our thanks to our partners and our children for their forbearance while we struggled to complete this self-imposed task. Now, perhaps we can also acknowledge how important their criticism as well as their support was to the emergence of the book.

In revising the text for the second edition some years later, we would like particularly to record our thanks to Kate Mosse for her useful and encouraging suggestions; and – for undertaking the daunting task of updating the medical chapters – Gill Yudkin, Fran Reader and Kirsten Duckitt, whose commitment to improving the conditions for women's well-being is evident in their meticulous, thorough and thoughtful contributions.

Although individual contributors' accounts speak for themselves, we accept, as editors, the responsibility for the opinions expressed in the book and its collective 'voice'.

Valerie Hey
Catherine Itzin
Lesley Saunders
Mary Anne Speakman

April 1995

Preface to the Second Edition

Lesley Saunders

> Pain. Pain. Pain. Is it ever going to stop?
> What did I do wrong?
> Is there anybody there?

When Valerie wrote to the *Women's Research and Resources Centre Newsletter* (as it was then), it was to see if there was indeed anyone there:

> A lone feminist trying to make sense of her recent miscarriage at 22 weeks would like to hear from other women who would like to share their personal experiences – with a possible view to publishing such stories.

WRRC Newsletter 6, 1980

Many women wrote back (so long ago, it now seems). There were lots of us 'there', unhappy, desperate, recuperating, wondering ... Addresses and telephone numbers were exchanged; grief and the beginnings of release shared. Some of us decided to meet each other; and out of those meetings, by a long and sometimes difficult route, came the first edition of this book.

When we started writing the book in the early 1980s, it was in the heady atmosphere of a common catharsis of bereavement, of personal revelation and collective discovery; intense and powerful but not wholly communicable. As we went on, we realised we wanted to produce the kind of book we wish we could have read. We would have wanted three things: *confirmation* that none of us was necessarily alone or abnormal in losing a baby nor in responding to this in the ways we each did; *information*, about our bodies, about miscarriage and ectopic pregnancy, about the structure and informing principles of the health services, about mourning and its complex individual processes; *affirmation* that we, individually and together, can do something positive – whether by understanding something we previously hadn't, or by finally allowing ourselves to grieve fully and freely, or by taking action for some kind of change.

It is a book with much pain in it. A book about miscarriage and ectopic pregnancy, about 'when things go wrong', which glossed over grief and terror would, for most women, have missed the heart of the experience. But one that stopped in the thick of the pain would very likely immobilise its readers by inviting them to read and share others' afflictions on top of their own without alerting them to the dynamic of recovery and change. So we have included both testimony and discussion which take us beyond the confines of the event which caused the pain.

The structure of the book reflects a generalised chronology of process; first, the loss, in 'Inside Stories'; then the need to gather and consider information, in 'Medical Viewpoints'; next, the construction and confirmation of a meaning, in 'Key Issues'; finally, affirmation, in 'Coming Through and Going On', that we can go on and through loss into a different place.

A reader might well therefore use this book to grieve with, at the time of loss or retrospectively – as we have done many times in its compilation. Then, as we also did, the reader can move on, slowly perhaps, but gaining comprehension and confidence.

We were worried that a notion seemed to have become popular in some quarters that miscarriage had been ignored by the women's movement because feminists preferred issues such as abortion which could be sloganised. Attitudes have perhaps changed in the years since 1989 when this book was first published, though feminism and feminists continue to be (deliberately) misunderstood. We felt, and still feel, that – contrary to such notions – it is important to continue the meticulous feminist practice of putting women's own words at the heart of health education. True to feminist theory also, the book tries to bring fresh analysis to bear on particular experiences common to women's lives – an experience in this instance characterised by a confused array of assertion and disputation by medical professionals and lay people alike, usually bolstered from behind with unargued assumptions about women and their social role.

Accordingly, we are concerned at some points to illuminate connections between things which are often polarised. We include, for example, alongside miscarriage and ectopic pregnancy, an account of abortion. We show the falsity of assuming that these experiences not only must be mutually opposed ethically and politically, but must also carry contrasting emotional charges. Women are subject to all kinds of pressures on their procreativity, ranging from inadequate contraception and lack of appropriate housing and childcare provision to sexual harassment and violence. In making space to grieve over their miscarried babies, women do not have to forfeit – for themselves or anyone else – the right at other times and places to make deliberate, difficult choices.

The other major disjunction which we attempt to re-connect is that between our present and future experiences as potential childbearers and our past experience as babies, foetuses ourselves. What does it mean to be a survivor of a threatened miscarriage and to be able, through a process of rediscovery, to recall that trauma? What are the implications of this information for parenting a child who is still in the womb, even one who may never be born?

In other places we make distinctions between things that are frequently bundled together, such as when we analyse, briefly, the compound meanings of motherhood. Neither wishing nor being able to duplicate the impressive and varied feminist contribution in this area, we nonetheless point out how disentangling the assumptions, institutions and expectations out of which 'motherhood' is constructed can be a crucial element in making sense of prebirth loss.

Other silences ought to be broken, although, because of the way our writing emerged from our support group, we have not done so here. Are there, for instance, further meanings of miscarriage for lesbians, for black women and women of colour or for disabled women, to which we have not been able to do full justice? We regret these omissions and look forward to other books written from those different perspectives.

We could tell you a story about the production of this book: during its middle phases it became extremely difficult to compile. The material had largely been written, but the book refused somehow to be viable. Work grew stilted; relationships faltered. It almost miscarried, you might say, as if at some obscure, collective level we still could not believe in our capacity to be effective, to bring a project to fruition. We had more work to do before the book could emerge – the subjective work of letting go and risking.

Reflecting now on those processes, as we bring the book up-to-date for its second edition, is quite strange. Many of the earlier emotional contours have been smoothed and flattened simply by the fact that – as lives and relationships change, careers progress or take u-turns or our longed-for babies become witty, scornful, loving, irritating and huge teenagers and then leave us – priorities inevitably change too. Our preoccupations have – for many of us and in what seems an astonishingly short time – taken a totally new form as we cope with menopause and the not-so-distant prospect of 'retirement'. Personally, I give four cheers for my own and my colleagues' greater sense of stability and confidence as the middle-aged women we are. But I also know that this sense has grown out of the rawness and depth of those other experiences on which this new version of the book, revised with great love and respect for our former selves, depends.

April 1995

Note: Medical and technical terms appearing in the text are explained either as they occur or, if used more than once, in the *Glossary* (Appendix 3).

Part One:
Inside Stories

Introduction

The following stories are a collection of individual experiences which, despite their significant differences, represent the material from which a narrative wholeness is plotted.

This collective story creates new understandings which displace the divisions which normally characterise the orthodoxy in thought about who women are and what women feel. This story challenges the taken-for-granted opposition between women who have elected to end their pregnancy and those who suffer birth loss involuntarily.

We fundamentally reject the notion that the concept of choice is more salient here than the continuities in grief and pain which unite us. Our analysis therefore puts together Lesley's account of her decision to abort her fourth child with Mary Anne's account of the loss of her first through the surgery necessitated by the child's conception as ectopic.

The analysis which is made from this perspective is a radical refusal to set up categories of good or bad mothers. It is about the making of a continuum which embraces all of us and allows us to name our world.

It is also important to specify however who the 'us' in this instance represents. These inside stories are *ours* and as such they are neither representative, comprehensive, or definitive testaments. They only tell our stories which are those of white, privileged, highly educated women. This is not offered as an apology; rather it is an expression of our taking responsibility fully for owning the truths they contain.

But ownership is not to be confused with possessiveness. These accounts are thus placed as central to this book as an invitation to other women to name their own world too.

It is only through this shared process of developing insights through open collective enterprise that this book has itself emerged to see the light of day. We offer these hard-won truths in celebration of this achieved solidarity. We hope these inside stories and their explanation speak to you too.

Valerie's Poem

Written about two weeks after her
miscarriage

Stars of the silent screen
Being groomed for success
A partnership. Duet
With me as your agent
Encouraging your growth
Unpromising beginnings
Very green; very new
Unsettled, fragile.

How we nursed your voices
One was always stronger than
The other;
Supervised your diets,
Appointments.
Measured your maturation
Precisely.

But all our care couldn't
Save you.
One of you insisted on a
Premature launching
Dragging the other behind
Reluctantly.

The limelight was waiting
You were sick of the dark
But you weren't ready
You weren't fully formed
Under-rehearsed amateurs
Second-rate, mediocre
You didn't have a chance.

Few came to your opening night
Me out of necessity
G because I made him
The others out of professionalism

But we all knew it'd be a
Non-event.

Why didn't you wait!
For the proper setting.
You blew it . . .

Valerie Hey

Lesley's Story

Before I'd had either a miscarriage or an abortion I never imagined them happening to me; but especially abortion. I marched on that NAC rally when the police stood guard outside Mothercare in London's West End. We scoffed at the notion behind this bizarre deployment of law officers – that women who support women's choice must feel violent towards the idea of motherhood, or even babies. We shouted 'Not the Church and not the State! Women shall decide our fate!' It didn't occur to me then that I could be one of the women I was marching for. Abortion was still something that happened to other people. I used to say that I supported the choice for other women but I wouldn't contemplate it for myself.

Now I realise that the miscarriage I had, the two children I bore and the abortion I chose were part of the same continuum which we are taught to see fragmented, in conflict: that complex unity of a woman's relationship to her biology, her creativity and her society.

There are many who would still divide us from ourselves, each other and our knowledge.

My daughter was born on the eve of the spring equinox. When she was born, I said, 'Now my life will change. I do not yet know how, only that there is a fizz in the air which means things will not go on as before.' Her birth was the whirlwind. About the only things that didn't change were my name and address. Before she was born, I felt myself to be wandering in a dry place where nothing moved. My son, my firstborn, was intensely precious to me, but his existence was a great responsibility. There were days, slow and heavy, when looking after us both seemed far beyond me. He and I are linked by our sameness; she and I by our differences. She is my Kore, the one I had to visit an underworld – of despair and aridity – to find. She brought the spring into my life, our lives, and things have not gone on as before. These children, boy and girl, grow – as all healthy, lucky ones do – way beyond their mother's expectations. Teeth fall; faces elongate. My son is a writer of stories and verses; my daughter is a builder of fantasy machines and elaborate dens.

When she was two, I became pregnant again. It was a bad year. My father died in the spring. I decided to have an abortion. I felt

I did not have the resources, physical or emotional, to raise another child.

For me, whose other children before their births had mapped the inner landscapes of reality with their quite definite dimensions, there was no question but that abortion was killing. I knew that, as I knew I had to make peace with this child I did not want. Other women may think and feel differently. I promised her – both M and I felt the child to be female – that her life-spark would somehow re-enter mine, I would take responsibility for carrying through the meaning of her life. I would dedicate my creative life to her because she had given up her life for me, in order that I could mother myself instead of her.

The decision was hard to make. I can't imagine a woman for whom it would be easy, despite insinuations by anti-abortionists. The children I have were not the children of this one's father. He and I would probably never have a child together if it wasn't this one. We were both nearing 40. We were sharing looking after his one and my two, we knew what being parents meant. We wanted and did not want to be immersed in that experience again. Indeed, that ambivalence caused me to conceive – I hadn't been as meticulous about contraception as if I'd been quite sure I wanted no more children.

In the early weeks of pregnancy, while the pregnancy test still showed negative, though I knew it to be false, I had time to feel this new being and to love her. I didn't tell my children, but held them close to me so the baby inside could feel them through my skin.

M was away. When he came back, I told him. Then began the difficult time, the time for action. I made an appointment at one of the well-known independent pregnancy advice centres based in London. I didn't even think of going to my GP. I believe now, having spoken to other women, that I needn't have been so pessimistic about the local NHS. My GP visited me for the aftercare and was careful to be sympathetic.

The people at the advice centre did what they should. A counsellor spent much time ascertaining whether my decision was a firm one made in knowledge of alternatives. She lectured me about future contraception. I remember her with respect, though without other emotion. After all, I was holding back most of mine, believing they would prejudice my chances if I revealed them. I knew that my decision was final and that I would regret it deeply. That was, and is, my prerogative. I took care from then on to gather my friends round me. M and I held each other often, feeling the baby there between us. We cried in each other's arms. I booked a place for a post-abortion workshop at the Women's Therapy Centre. I visited a healer the evening before the abortion.

We drove through a beautiful early morning to the clinic in a leafy London suburb. The sun shone brilliantly, kindly, as we woke to what was happening. It was September. I had just had my thirty-seventh birthday. We parted – he would come for me later. This time I wasn't dismayed to be alone. I had to prepare myself and the baby: I needed the time.

Here is part of what I wrote that day:

Before the abortion

> I commit you, baby, to the elements
> I let you go into the world beyond
> I dedicate your life and my creativeness to each other
> I cast my love for M, and his for me, adrift from the moorings
> of childbearing.

> I am frightened – the place is unfamiliar. I'm trying to let go into the energy of life, feeling small, not hanging on.

> Heal my baby, heal, go well. Your spirit is getting ready to fly.

After the abortion

> Oh, the pain and tears are for later. For now, I am glad to be here and well, and relatively undrugged – though my pupils are tremendously dilated; probably the Valium. I took one tablet and hid the other; wanted to feel woozy but not mindless: I reckoned that though I might be dulled on the physical level and to some extent emotionally by those 5 mgs, still the intuitive level would be open and energetic. I'm taking the [homeopathic] remedies Elizabeth gave me last night.

I'd requested a local anaesthetic; the doctor agreed, after I'd persisted. I felt that I wanted to be as awake while the baby was leaving me as I was when she was conceived. I'm not sure the doctor agreed with my logic – she was more concerned that I'd be able to 'cope'. I realised afterwards that the relative autonomy I had and the sympathy I felt from staff were, in part, due to my 'status' – mother of two, in a stable relationship, late thirties, well educated ... I don't mean women were in general unkindly treated; it was just that hint of 'silly girls!' in the nurses' attitudes. They intended no harm, but no respect either. We'd have to jolly well pull up our socks in future.

It was painful and shocking. Not as painful as birth, but sharper, and where I couldn't get it. I just kept saying, 'Bye bye baby, bye bye baby,' letting the pain out in soft moans as the instruments went in and, after an age, came out again. Afterwards I lay curled in the recovery room like a foetus myself, full of hurt.

The doctor had remonstrated with me once before the operation that it wasn't a 'baby'. Perhaps she didn't want me to upset myself, or perhaps she didn't want to upset herself. That would be quite comprehensible. As is pointed out elsewhere in the book, terminology plays a big part in mystifying pregnancy loss; but it is also a protection of sorts for doctors in dealing, unsupported, with their own distress in difficult work.

As usual, my womb is bulky. They say I was ten weeks pregnant but they had to dilate me for twelve. I believe my womb has tended to be enlarged, too open – as after the miscarriage and in the post-partum haemorrhage with Leon's birth – because I couldn't acknowledge its reality in my life. But now I want it to be smaller, less of a portal through which the whole of life's meaning comes and goes. I want its energy to be diffused. So close now, my womb, find peace in a smaller space. Let us be friends.

I am dispersed, scattered, after all these changes of self into other, my flesh into other flesh, other substance. Writing is an act of collection, of gathering the fragments. Of putting stones in a basket and watching for them to turn into bread.

Or, writing out of a place of no-place. Spinning one's substance into words, living off one's own flesh. Writing the history of events separated by years and false assumptions into a story with a unified meaning. Writing out of a death, a desert, a stony place, making it blossom.

Very close to the fourth anniversary of this baby's death, *Glancing Fires*, the book I compiled on women's creativity, was published. I had laboured on it in what I understood as an enaction of my promise: it contains the work and visions of twenty women poets, painters, dancers, singers, creators. It is dedicated to her.

In one sense and for me, it *is* her. This is the month, as I write, of warm flowery days and frosty nights when she would have been three. Sometimes in the dark with M inside me I can feel the place where she was and it makes me cry. Whether the tears are grief or something quite different, I can't say.

Mary Anne's Story

Mary Anne had an ectopic pregnancy at ten weeks. It was her first baby.

My second period didn't come – I really must be pregnant. Next week I'll go to the doctor. But then two days into what would have been my period, I went into town to do some shopping and started having abdominal cramps. When I got home, I found I'd been bleeding, just a very little, but still blood.

I remember going into the garden and looking at the spring flowers coming into bud. My next door neighbour came out and started to talk about how my garden had looked many years before – a scene engraved on my memory. I thought how inconsequential this conversation was when something inside me was going wrong.

I went indoors and phoned the doctor's surgery. The receptionist was kind and said I should come round at the beginning of the afternoon surgery. When I went, my doctor was also sympathetic, scolded me for having come and said I should go straight home to bed and that my husband should take round a specimen of urine in the morning. I spent three days in bed, still a little spotting and some cramps. I phoned the surgery – the specimen was contaminated by the blood so they didn't know whether I was pregnant. I was told to take things easy and phone if the bleeding continued.

The bleeding and cramps stopped. Was everything going to be all right? All the other signs of pregnancy were still there and becoming even more noticeable. But it was very difficult to carry on as 'normal'. My whole consciousness was swamped by a big question mark. By this time I'd told a couple of close women friends and I was glad of their support; was very glad I'd told them when, later, things really did go wrong.

About ten days after this the cramps came back with a vengeance. I phoned the surgery again and once again went round. This time I explicitly asked if it might be an ectopic pregnancy – I'd known of someone who'd had one and the symptoms were similar; the cramps were not like period pains but specifically on one side – the right in my case. Yes, it might be. An appointment was made to attend the antenatal clinic at the hospital there and then. Back home, my husband drove me to the clinic and came in with me.

After about an hour (it felt like six), I was finally put in a cubicle, on a couch and waited for the doctor. He finally came and went through all the questions again: why am I here; what are my dates. 'Oh, well, it's a bit early for a first visit.' 'Yes, but I've been bleeding and I've got these pains in my side. My GP thought it best to check . . .' 'Oh . . . Do you want to be pregnant?' 'Yes, I do.' (And it's not a phantom pregnancy, which I can see you think it is; it's not all in my imagination – it's real, I've had other signs.) 'We don't have a positive urine test.' 'But you can't be sure; my breasts are tender and bigger; my sleep pattern's changed,' etc. etc. Silently, 'Why won't you listen to me, to what my body is saying?'

It was finally decided to do an ultrasound (see pp. 115–16). The X-ray department was at the other end of the hospital; then a long, draughty wait by the porter's entrance. Change into another, flimsier gown, behind a screen that anyone passing could see through. The ultrasound didn't show anything – the radiographer kept giving me more water to drink, but it still didn't show anything. The doctor came in and he had a look, still unsuccessful. 'Might it be in the tube?' he queried – so I knew he *had* thought of this which was some comfort. But they couldn't tell. This moment was awful – I knew I was pregnant but the baby was nowhere to be found.

Some years later, my GP arranged for me to have a hysterosalpingogram X-ray, which is to look at the condition of the uterus and fallopian tubes. Before I went to have the X-ray I had a dream which I believe is very firmly related to the ultrasound experience. In the dream I visited my GP to get the results of the X-ray and she said the X-ray had been inconclusive because they couldn't find my fallopian tube.

Anyway, the ultrasound was also inconclusive and the doctor was puzzled. Finally he said he didn't think it was an ectopic pregnancy (though he didn't say why) but that if I was in fact pregnant, it was possible that I might be about to have an 'ordinary miscarriage'. I should phone if anything else happened. By this time, I think he'd picked up my feeling of panic and had assumed a perfect example of the reassuring bedside manner. Except I actually felt far from reassured.

This all happened on a Friday. The pains continued, but less intensely, the next day. On Sunday I woke feeling well again, no pains, no bleeding – I allowed myself to hope again. We went for a long walk by the sea – it was beautiful and sunny.

On Monday morning, I woke feeling sick and couldn't even drink a cup of tea. L went off to his office. I stayed in bed. From nine a.m. to four p.m. the day passed in a state of semi-coma. I had constant pain in my side, I vomited, I passed out for a while. I was unable to get to the phone – to do that would have been to admit I needed help, that this time, things really were wrong. But by the time L got back at four o'clock I knew this couldn't continue. I got downstairs and phoned the hospital. I must have sounded hysterical because the telephonist wouldn't believe I wanted the antenatal ward but wanted to put me through to the labour ward. When I got through, I had to explain it all to the sister who hadn't been there on Friday, but she said I should come straight in.

At the hospital I was taken by wheelchair to a ward and helped/lifted into a bed. By this time I was very weak and felt very faint. L went out to park the car properly and it was ages before I saw him again. A houseman came and we went through all the questions again. And then an internal examination – this was one of the most horrific things I've ever been through. He didn't want to add to my pain like this. When the registrar came, the first doctor argued strongly, and, thank God, successfully, for me not to have another internal. The result of this, in terms of diagnosis, was either an ectopic pregnancy or an ovarian cyst.[1]

The outcome, in practical terms, was to attach me to a drip and transfer me by ambulance to the main hospital where the gynaecology department was situated. I briefly saw L before this happened, not enough time to give each other the support we both needed.

The doctors explained that I would have a laparoscopy to see what was going on, and, if necessary, a laparotomy (see pp. 104–106). The operation took place at eight p.m. When I came round, at about five a.m., my first action was to feel my abdomen. Yes, there was a load of padding, sticky from blood, and it hurt like hell. I must have called out because two nurses came over. I asked what had happened – had it been an ectopic pregnancy? They didn't know. Can you please find out? One of them went to look at my notes and came back to tells me, yes, it had been. My right tube and its tiny baby had been removed.

Valerie's Story

Valerie miscarried twins at 22 weeks.

The actual physical events followed an almost morbidly predictable course: at about 20 weeks I fell down some stairs, 12 in all, and badly bruised myself as well as being terrified of the potential consequences. Nothing happened immediately. I phoned the doctor and asked for advice but I had no cramping or blood loss.

A week later during the night I was disturbed by severe pain in my stomach which I dismissed as 'wind'. It was severe enough to get me out of bed and had gone by the morning. I didn't see it as an indicator of a 'threatened' miscarriage so I carried on as normal, planning my journey to Manchester via Newbury and Nottingham. We were going to fly from Manchester Airport for a holiday in Canada and the USA.

The first sign that made me take action was a slight blood loss in Newbury before we were due to depart from Nottingham. I phoned the local clinic, who advised rest – they said I should lie in the back of the car with my feet up, which is what I did for the whole journey.

It was at my friend's house that my membranes ruptured and I was admitted as an emergency to Nottingham Maternity Hospital, where I was first examined by the consultant, and later by another doctor, before being placed on the women's surgical ward. It is quite apparent to me that I was an administrative problem, i.e. where do they put a woman who is threatening to miscarry? The fact that I was moved twice indicates that they were responding to my sensitivities and situation – in other words, the staff didn't just send me to maternity immediately.

The 'solution' of holding me in a ward full of post-operative women was hardly adequate – it was traumatic seeing these women who had just had hysterectomies and who were in great pain. I didn't exactly sleep that night locked in as I was with my own anxiety. No one can tell you whether you will miscarry and in my case I spent eight days in the place, still leaking amniotic fluid, before the situation went beyond the point of no return.

The anguish and distress I went through cannot be described. I had superb nursing. The 'doctoring'[1] was much less personal and no one seemed able to supply me with any answers. Each person seemed to have their own theories, some more positive than others. The truth is no one would predict the outcome.

After the first two days, when I had an ultrasound scan to see that the foetuses were still being sustained by sufficient fluid, I was admitted to the maternity unit proper. This was a purpose-built attractive small-ward, three-floor building.

Needless to say, I was placed on the ward/floor with other women experiencing obstetric difficulties, ranging from high blood pressure to Caesarian section, breech presentation, toxaemia and other 'abnormal' conditions. Each day I was monitored: blood pressure taken, foetal heart monitoring, temperature, urine, blood samples, etc. All of which focused my full attention on my womb; the nurses referred to my womb's contents as 'babies' and especially since I was carrying twins their 'humanity' became more real to me at the same time as it was being scrutinised for its possible erasure. This contradiction must surely lie at the heart of the experience.

On the Friday, ten days after being admitted, I just felt too miserable to get up for breakfast (on all other occasions I managed to do this when I wasn't on bed rest); I lay on my bed and wept.

The consultant came on his rounds at one p.m. and in an internal examination saw that a cord from one of the foetuses had come down the cervix; he couldn't hear a foetal heart beat of one of the twins and so the inevitable decision was taken to induce an abortion because of the risk of infection. There was no possibility of operating via a Caesarian to save the other – being twins made each foetus much smaller than a corresponding single pregnancy; anyway the minimum age for foetal survival is 24 weeks.[2] All this I'd been told quite early on in my hospitalisation. The unit was equipped with every technological back-up service, i.e. special care baby unit specifically designed for premature or difficult births, but the gestation age of my pregnancy was just too immature to use their facilities.

Early on during my stay on the gynaecological ward I'd noted my womb stretching and tightening and obviously these were weak contractions which I refused to admit because I didn't want to recognise the significance of the admission.

The process began at three p.m. and lasted until ten p.m. I was treated with care, respect and extreme sympathy by the midwife sister in charge. She talked to me about pain relief and left the decision about that to me.

At no time did she treat me just as a 'case' – I was a woman who was dealing with an event on numerous different levels. She did offer me tremendous support and her competence and warm personality helped me cope. My lover was there all the time, too, and he was also superb – I really felt that he was *with* me. The midwife asked me numerous questions throughout the labour, e.g. did I want to see them; did I want them to be sent for tests to the histology lab?

She left the power in my hands – vitally important, when I was feeling that my body was out of control, to gain a sense of dignity and strength from being encouraged to decide on these issues. She recognised how important it was for me to feel that I could find something positive in all this trauma. Despite the pain, and the mental pain of going through a process which I knew would have no live products at the end, I managed to secure from the situation a new type of knowledge about myself – a centre of inner courage and strength. I know it sounds self-centred but I had to find a meaning for the event – I had to make it into a source of learning about myself.

I know other women may find it a strange line of thought and would have wanted to be drugged during the course of the labour, but I managed to salvage a sense of my own force by remaining fully conscious and lucid throughout the time. It was near the end, I realise, when I sent my lover off to find the sister (she'd gone off to aid another woman nearby) to give me some pain relief. By then I was sufficiently dilated for the final expulsions to occur.

I didn't see the babies; my lover did. The nurse told me how their little eyes were closed. The midwife said that to her eyes and G's eyes they were twin boys.

Afterwards I was just glad to be out of pain – the relief was tremendous. I felt that I'd achieved something – my unconscious mind registered this too. I was in a state of shock for weeks after, I now realise, being too numb to really cry. I recall feeling anxious on leaving the hospital – a tremendous feeling of 'leaving something behind'; I didn't want to go until I'd found it. There was a ritual of shedding flower petals – a carnation – which I sprinkled out of my window.

My wretched body let me know that it had prepared itself for pregnancy by producing vast quantities of milk three days later. This was itself another physical/emotional crisis – the doctor or nurses should have given me a milk depressant before I left the place. I think the pharmacy was closed on Sunday, so I never received the medication.

Sheila's Story

Sheila's second pregnancy ended in a miscarriage at 11 weeks.

Second pregnancy – n⁄ problems – felt great – no sickness. Continued playing sq. ;h and mountaineering although at a reduced pace. Went to Snowdonia mountaineering with a friend for a long weekend at 11 weeks. Took things easy, carried reduced weights but had three good days on the hills. Returned Sunday evening. Monday felt tired but to be expected. Did little all day – my turn to look after Paul (first child, then 16 months), but he was no trouble. A visitor for tea which P [partner] was cooking. I went to have a quick bath before eating – noticed some bleeding. The first sign of any trouble. I panicked immediately – felt totally shocked – called P – didn't even feel able to go down two flights of stairs to tell him.

I knew immediately that I would lose the baby. It was the first moment after the full-term pregnancy and 11 weeks of the present pregnancy that I felt scared that something could go, and in fact now was going, wrong. The possibility of problems had never before occurred to me. I knew things could go wrong in pregnancy but I felt I was the one of the lucky ones who would sail through it with very little alteration from the norm (apart from getting bigger!). I was totally shattered. I was someone whose life revolved around bodily activity. I had worked hard to gain control in body action, to be aware of how my body moved and reacted to stimuli. I was fit and healthy. Now I felt I had lost all control of my body. I kept bleeding and there was nothing I could do about it. It was the first feelings of guilt (feelings that were to remain with me for a long time) – that I of all people should be experiencing something other than a normal pregnancy. 'Pregnancy is not an illness'; you should be able to continue as before with slight limitations. I, who enjoyed fitness and activity, was now faced with terrible guilt. Had I brought on this miscarriage myself? Oh, why had I been so selfish to go away the weekened before? I had felt the need for a break so had naturally gone to the mountains. I must have overstrained myself – it was my fault. If only . . .

These initial reactions continued. P called for the doctor immediately and I reached for some support from my health books.

I received very little. The doctor was involved in his evening surgery and said he would call round as soon as he finished.

The doctor arrived soon after seven p.m. (not my doctor but a partner). He was very pleasant, quite sympathetic but very matter of fact. There was nothing he could do – my body was now in control. He said that it was *extremely* common to bleed at this stage in pregnancy – it usually simply stopped itself. However if I was to get any pain and/or blood clots I was to let him know immediately. He suggested rest but said that there was no need to stay in bed. His whole approach was fatalistic – what was to be would happen, regardless of any attempted interventions from him. He said that he had stopped even examining women in this situation as he was sure it was of no help and in fact could simply make matters worse. I found his attitude reassuring, as a doctor's honesty about his inability to help seemed refreshing. However, I was still convinced I was losing the baby and found it *very* difficult to relax.

I had similar bleeding (equivalent to a period) for 24 hours. It didn't appear to worsen so I was in a continual state of waiting for something to happen. The most distressing aspect was that I had little idea of what I could expect to happen. I found this to be the most terrifying part of the whole miscarriage. How did one actually lose a baby? *Our Bodies, Ourselves* talked most frighteningly about 'bleeding and cramping lasting a few days sometimes starting and stopping regularly, *until the contents are completely expelled*' (emphasis added). Then even more distressingly:

> The foetus, amniotic sac and placenta, along with a lot of blood, may be expelled completely intact. You'll probably know when this is happening. It's very important to say here that if you are not in a hospital you must do the difficult task of collecting the foetus and afterbirth and putting it in a clean container, and taking it to the hospital for the laboratory to examine.[1]

I just couldn't imagine coping with the above situation. I, who was trained in first aid and prepared to cope with any situation in an outdoor accident, just could not comprehend the thought of actually producing a partially developed foetus – our future baby. I kept saying to myself, 'Please let me be in hospital when it finally happens.' I was still not sure how much it was a gradual process or whether there was the equivalent of a birth. This terrible fear was the most powerful and distressing part of the ordeal and remained with me until I had eventually been into hospital and had had a D and C. I think, also, I must stress how important I felt it was not to be left alone at any time from that initial onset of bleeding. I felt so scared and vulnerable that I really needed the support of having someone continually with me, both during those first stages and later in hospital.

The final stage of the miscarriage began about 24 hours after the initial signs. I was not unduly surprised, for, as I have said, I was convinced that I was losing the baby. I began to have cramping pain, as with a period, and I noticed slight clotting in my discharge. P went to call a doctor. There was no question of waiting, as I felt I must get into hospital before *it* happened. We had no phone, so P had to go out to ring. As usual there was no one available but he eventually got a locum. He had to go out on another call but would come later. He saw no urgency in the situation! By P's return I had started to bleed very heavily. The blood was now bright red (as opposed to the previous dark red loss). I felt that I was simply emptying my whole contents. The pains worsened and became more like the contractions of labour. I felt totally incapable of moving. Again it was *the fear of the unknown*. What was going to happen when . . .? Meanwhile we tried to maintain calm for our little boy, who obviously didn't know what was happening. P got him ready for bed and took him to a neighbour. This itself was made more traumatic as we had only lived here for two months so were new to the neighbourhood. We waited. No doctor came. My contractions were now very painful and quite regular and I was bleeding heavily.

P took the decision and went out yet again. This time he called an ambulance who at first refused to come as they need a doctor's authorisation! They were given little choice by P and within a short time arrived. I can remember quite vividly the ambulancemen – they were extremely calm and rather disbelieving as to whether anything much was happening! They took my pulse, which was fairly high, understandably, and commented that I must be getting myself into a bit of a state! I felt they were extremely con-descending. All I wanted to do was to go and get it over with. 'How do you know she is miscarrying?' they asked P. By then I was fairly well covered in blood as sanitary towels were of little use. His reply was equally scathing. So I was put into the ambulance at last, having convinced them that I did need admitting to hospital. As we drove away, the doctor arrived! He looked quite astonished and it seems commented that I must have been the first patient that he had admitted to hospital without ever even meeting. A comment perhaps on the whole system of medical availability and help. I had to go alone to hospital. I would have dearly loved P to be with me for support and to fight any battles which would no doubt be inevitable in dealing with the hospital process. However, my priority was that he must stay with our son.

The journey is hazy now. I was in considerable pain. I was admitted and left to await examination. The pains were worse and I was fighting to control them and myself. Remember your relaxation I told myself. But I had little will or encouragement to relax and do my breathing exercises learned from my first labour. This time I knew that there was to be no joyous end to the pain. I was still unsure what to expect.

Eventually a doctor arrived and after an extremely painful internal examination gave me some painkillers. He said something about whether I knew I was miscarrying. Did I know I was pregnant? He seemed to remove several large blood clots and I felt slightly better in terms of the pain. He then said that I needed a D and C and would in fact try to get theatre time as soon as possible rather than wait until morning. Thank God! I had fought to remain calm throughout. I was determined not to seem hysterical. I find it hard to divulge my feelings at the best of times. It was in those next few seconds that the truth hit me hard for the first time. After all this waiting – about 36 hours – it was nearly all over. For the first time I realised that although I had been convinced I would lose the baby, I had always held on to that last vestige of hope. Now that was gone. I silently cried.

I had my D and C at about one a.m., after quite a wait by the operating theatre. However, I had had a pre-op injection so everything was relatively hazy about this time and I was quite relaxed. I remember being moved around and being returned to a side room by a ward for the rest of the night. I was on a drip and they woke me frequently to take my blood pressure. It all now seems to be almost dreamlike, the clarity of the memory fading with time. I do remember lying there knowing it was all over. It was a foul night – the rain was hammering against the window. It all seemed so unreal. I felt absolutely no emotion at that point – I just wanted to go home.

I was discharged in the morning with a bottle of iron tablets and some antibiotics to help avoid infection. This was the sum total of any aftercare by the medical profession – my case was now closed.

Phil's Story

We thought that it was very important to include in this section a male partner's account of his thoughts upon the miscarriage which his wife went through. So often is the notion of masculinity set up as the opposite to femininity that male responsibilities and involvement with respect to the growth and loss of children are ignored. The following account is some acknowledgment of this need to open up the subject for male partners too.

Throughout Sheila's first pregnancy and for the first 11 weeks of her second she had virtually no problems. She had been very fit and active. Sheila had been to the mountains with a friend for a long weekend.

On the Monday evening I was cooking when I heard her call from upstairs. Although she sounded quite calm, I could tell from the tone in her voice that something was wrong. She had started to bleed and I could tell that she was sure it was serious. Even after the doctor had examined her and had told her that bleeding at this stage often happened it was clear that Sheila thought the pregnancy was about to end.

There was nothing physical that could be done except to wait and to make sure that Sheila was – as far as was possible in the circumstances – comfortable. I had been to pregnancy classes with her but there was nothing that we had read, seen or heard which helped us to face the possibility of a loss.

Relaxation was impossible for her; she started to question what *she* had done. The problem is that in situations like this you can see that rationally there is no cause-and-effect but emotionally it is hard to accept. We tried to exorcise all emotions of blame – an all but impossible objective when women are so regularly held responsible for any problems, no matter how minor, relating to childbirth, children or the family.

We went through the next 24 hours without any idea of what was happening or what might happen. As the bleeding continued, I began to realise that the pregnancy might end quickly. I prepared myself mentally to handle that situation if it happened suddenly.

There was no consideration at this time for 'the baby' – as far as I was concerned it did not exist – my only worry was for Sheila. I knew I had to convince myself that I would cope because if it happened quickly I would be the only person there other than Sheila.

Later on the Tuesday it became clear that Sheila was about to lose the baby. As soon as Sheila said that she was getting cramp and 'this was it', there could be no doubt in my mind. There is no way that anyone else can judge or decide what is happening more accurately than the person herself.

I ran to the phone to get the doctor – I rang the fourth number – the call was re-directed and I got the stand-by doctor. I told him, as quietly and fully as I could, Sheila's symptoms and the developments of the previous 24 hours.

He said, in his distant wisdom, that there was no emergency. He was speaking from his office over ten miles away and he said he would call 'later'. End of medical care!

I ran home and by now Sheila was bleeding heavily and in considerable pain. Within minutes she was having regular contractions and losing a lot of blood. She was in a lot of pain. I bathed her and tried to ease her pain but it was no use. There was no sign of the doctor. I dialled for an ambulance. They refused to come without a doctor's authorisation. This made me very angry and I told them to come immediately; as far as I was concerned the doctor might never come.

My persistence paid off – the ambulancemen arrived and immediately put me in my place. They clearly doubted that much was happening, despite Sheila's pain and the amount of blood. 'How do you know she's miscarrying?' was the first doubting question. 'There's no rush, don't panic – we don't want to take you in as well' was the follow up. Sheila's pain was obvious as they took her downstairs and put her in the ambulance.

They had just gone when the doctor turned up. He asked me to sign something – a document saying that he had made his visit and had called an ambulance. I told him what he could do with his form!

Friends turned up to give their support. The minute I saw them my feelings burst out and I cried on Mike's shoulder. Again the impact of what was happening focused solely on Sheila, what she was going through at the hospital – the clinical, sterilised, impersonal and masked routine of the operating theatre. I hoped against hope that someone would show her some warmth – put their arms around her to give her a shoulder to cry on.

The slightest show of her emotions would probably bring the

typical response to all women in real pain: 'Pull yourself together', or 'It can't be that bad'. Little did they know. At two a.m. they told me that she had been through theatre, had a D and C and was doing well.

That night in bed I lay and willed myself to be with her, sharing the pain and trying to help. Of course none of this was really relevant to her pain or to her feelings. Like childbirth and its pain, you can be supportive but you can't experience it – it's her body and, to that extent, her enclosed and very personal world.

I had been with Sheila throughout the long 17 hours of labour with Paul (our first child). There is so much nonsense talked about the 'wonderful physical experience' of the act of birth. For Sheila it was incredibly difficult and painful and much as I could help and sponge her face, it was not my body that went through the pain. At least Paul was there at the end of the tunnel – this time there was to be nothing, just emptiness and a deep sense of loss.

I collected Sheila from the hospital. I tried to make the journey as comfortable as possible with pillows and blankets. We talked quietly – there was a lot to say.

The loss hadn't really affected me. I was too tied into Sheila's physical condition and her feelings to think much about a 'baby' being 'lost'. The baby had no identity for me as such – it had not been in my body in that sense, so it was not 'there' – but Sheila was 'there' and was struggling to make sense of the previous 36 hours.

We arrived home and Sheila went to bed. She couldn't sleep, couldn't get comfortable and couldn't relax. My own personal feelings were dominated by a deep sense of my own inadequacy to help her. Eventually we came through but there were deep anxieties, not only about the loss but also about becoming pregnant again.

Although Sheila was soon fully fit and again very active, her next pregnancy was much less easy to handle. The worries and doubts returned and limited her physical activities, although everything went well.

There is no way that I felt, experienced or could touch the emotions that Sheila suffered in the loss of a baby. Obviously I was saddened and disappointed but that is nothing compared to what Sheila endured.

Marilyn's Story

Marilyn's third and fourth pregnancies ended in miscarriage at 13 and nine weeks. For a while it was thought that the second might be an ectopic pregnancy.

When I was pregnant for the third time and found that I was bleeding slightly at eight weeks I was quite alarmed. Nothing like this had ever happened before. I hoped desperately that it would stop. I had a quiet day. It was easy enough. We were on holiday. (It had not occurred to me before this moment of writing that I should have gone to the doctor then . . . but I was so accustomed to my body being 'ordinary', doing what I wanted of it.) I think my fear was stronger than the above word 'alarmed' lets on to. It probably blotted out the information I had read about what to do in such circumstances. It was like panic, but I think it must have been quite well repressed panic. And then . . . there was only one incident of bleeding . . . It stopped. And once it stopped I don't remember giving the incident much thought. I carried on as usual. Got on with living, working, enjoying the summer, looking forward to the baby.

Then I bled at 12 weeks too. This time it did not stop. I was at home. I rang the GP. I went to bed. I was prescribed pills that would stop the bleeding.[1] They did, almost. Everything seemed to turn on whether the bleeding stopped. The days went by. I was desperate that there would be no more . . . I had no real idea what was happening to me. I was 'threatening to miscarry' but the words actually had no meaning for me. I had no understanding of losing a baby.

The slight pink discharge had gone on for a week. I was beginning to feel edgy, to feel as though I was going to have to live with it (there was a sense in which it was not connected to an actual baby). I wasn't very happy, but at least I was still resting. I was hungry. I told myself that was a good thing. Feeling hungry must surely mean that I was still pregnant. I must be. I became more unhappy. I had to admit to myself that there were pains. Only small, like period pains. I told myself they would go away. They didn't. They became stronger. I don't know how long I lay there waiting, hoping for them to stop, but I remember that I suddenly changed. Suddenly I seemed to be filled with a kind of urgency. I wanted help, care, reassurance, information; I had to find out what was happening to me – and I didn't want to stay in that house any more.

At the hospital I was left in a large green-painted room on a high couch against one wall. I lay there alone. The pain came, regularly, I talked. I talked aloud. More frequently the pains came. I choked. I cried. My body was giving birth – and it was too soon, much too soon. I talked aloud. I cried for it to stop. I fought each pain as it came. It wasn't time for contractions. Not now! I tried to take my mind away from what my body was doing against my will; my eyes soaked in the detail of the cracks in the ceiling, the brushmarks in the paint on the wall, a dent in the plaster – and I wept, uncontrollably. The contractions grew stronger. In my head I shouted. I didn't want to give birth. But I could do nothing to stop what was happening. Nothing. Just cry.

Steadily and more painfully the contractions happened, and dementedly I cried. I cried against them. Eventually someone else came. (I realise now it was probably the night staff coming on duty). There was an air of efficiency. The fact that I was there suddenly mattered. They were going to move me. There was a gentle hand. My swollen face, my tear-stained self was accepted. I was taken up to the wards, into a side ward – en route I was given an injection. It would take away the pain, they seemed to say. My father came back again (he had to leave earlier). We talked – about other things. The injection had dulled the pain – and the pain in my heart too. I could no longer resist the weariness of my drugged body. My father left. The bed felt damp. I slept. I was slow to realise that the waters had broken the night before. That had never happened to me spontaneously before. I had woken up exhausted with crying, but crying still, more softly. I needed a bedpan. I felt vague and unreal. A nurse came with a bedpan. I explained that the waters seemed to have broken. She left me. I awoke to a reality that I had not understood. Miscarriage was this – a tiny, warm, baby that slipped – too easily – from my body, small, curled, into the bedpan.

The nurse came back. I said something facile, like, 'I think it's come out.' She lifted the bedpan away from beneath me. I put my hands out. I said, 'I want to look at it.' She didn't move any further, and I looked and looked – at the tiny arms, and fingers, the little curled shape, knees snuggled up against such a little body – toes, everything perfectly there – the sleeping foetal face. I wanted to touch it, pick it up – it was beautiful. It was mine. 'Was it a boy or a girl?' I asked her. She shook her head. Couldn't tell. I sensed that I could not pick it up in front of her, hold it in my hands – just a long, long look. She waited. And when she took it away it was because I said she could. It took me a long, long time to do that. It was a terrible thing to say, but I knew there was nothing else. It had to be goodbye. The nurses went. The tears came again. A deluge.

Some months later I became pregnant again. I felt happy, secretive about it (my usual feeling in early pregnancy) and after about the sixth week, slightly uneasy. I also felt rather unhealthy – and I smelt slightly wrong to myself (whether that's a relevant physical symptom I don't know – ignorance again).

At eight weeks I lost a small clot of blood in the lavatory. I was aghast. I didn't want to believe it. It just couldn't be true that the whole wretched thing was beginning again. However, I thought I knew better this time. I was going to take no risks. I went to bed. I didn't move. Dr Q came again (since I was registered with a panel of GPs it seemed sensible to ask for the same one. I clung to the notion that since he knew about the last miscarriage he would be better able to deal with this threat). He was matter of fact. There was no internal examination this time (I would have refused to have it had he suggested it), but a pregnancy test. I think he prescribed the same drug to stop bleeding – but I can't quite remember. That was the beginning of the week. Each day I lay there. I tried to keep calm. There was no alarming loss, only the slightest pink discharge. I waited and I hoped. Surely hope was justified this time.

There was something about the result of the pregnancy test that I couldn't grasp. Wouldn't my body behave as it had last time – would there be no contractions? And the foetus? (Dr Q didn't seem to know. He didn't seem to care.) It might have gone with that first (only) small clot of blood. But – I was confused. I had to make up the story for myself. Tell myself that nine weeks is not so far on as 13 weeks, that this time the foetus might have stopped growing even earlier. For me a timely and gentle explanation of the physical possibilities would, I think, have eased the anguish. Perhaps nobody could have known what happened – but to have talked about the *likelihood* of what had happened would have helped me in those first few hours. But perhaps I am alone in wanting to know the physical details.

The story is not at an end here, however. At the local general hospital I was examined by a doctor on admission; she was young,

female. I felt crushed, but having spent the whole afternoon in tears
I was no longer demented with grief. As I was examined a
tenderness revealed itself – just where the fallopian tube was – on
one side. She explained that the pregnancy might be ectopic. She
seemed to think that from all I had told her the possibility was real.
I could feel the pain. It was a reality that I could not deny. She
explained that an investigation would be necessary – a laparoscopy.
That was the only way of being certain. For that there would be a
small incision in my navel. If everything was all right, if the
pregnancy had been straightforward – then they would go ahead
simply with the D and C. I questioned her endlessly. The
physiological details? My chances of conceiving again with only
one fallopian tube? She answered patiently, and willingly. But the
pain was there – and the inevitability of the full-scale operation
seemed to be signalled by the pain. Sometimes you can pretend that
something does not hurt. (That's something you do as a child.) I
could not pretend to myself. A baby would no longer be so easy. I
would no longer be whole. Half of me was dying. That was how I
felt. I pressed the place myself. It was tender. There was no more
information I could ask her for.

My mind seems to have been numb after this. Except during the
examination, R [partner] had been with me. I have no recollection
of how he reacted, only that he was there, supportive, and gentle.
(He had been sad when I told him I was not pregnant.) There was
the routine of preparing for the operation. All I remember clearly
was hearing myself say, as the anaesthetic crept over me, 'All I
wanted was a baby.' In my head it seemed such a simple thing.

Out of darkness I spun through an unspeakably terrifying cosmic
dream/nightmare of trying to communicate through wires of time
and space and at the nightmare point I broke into the vagueness of
post-anaesthetic reality. My body was numb. There was a question
in my mind that had to be answered while oblivion seemed still
attainable. My hand moved across my tummy. There was nothing!
Smooth skin – no huge dressing. I remember feeling again. Stunned
into disbelief. There was nothing but a small piece of sticking
plaster over my navel. The anaesthetic disappeared. I came alive, I
was whole!

Ann's Story

Ann miscarried her first baby at eight weeks.

I could hardly believe it when I saw the bloodstains. I tried to dismiss them but worried and worried and finally rang my doctor. I was put through to a duty doctor and curtly told that it sounded as though I might be going to have a miscarriage but that this was not inevitable. 'Lie in bed and rest,' I was told, 'there is nothing else that can be done.' Frightened and alone I tried to ring N [partner], who was away from home, but couldn't get him, so finally I went to bed too shaken to sleep.

Early the next morning I called a friend. I needed to get some food but also I needed someone to talk to. She said she would rush round and, without asking, announced she was going to come and stay until things sorted themselves out. I was greatly relieved, for I was frightened not just of the idea that I might lose my child but also because I couldn't imagine what would happen. During the night I had already pored over *Our Bodies, Ourselves*[1] but that had not really told me what to expect. Meanwhile I still wanted to cling to the hope that everything would turn out well. Only two days before our decision had seemed to be whether to have a child or not, and now suddenly it all seemed out of control. There was nothing to be done except wait.

Over the next two days the fact that there *was* nothing that could be done was one of the hardest things to come to terms with. The bloodstains were slight and only occurred at intervals that were many hours apart. Each time they disappeared I clung to the hope that this time they would have gone for good. My cousin, who had had twins a few years before, had bled for several days in mid-pregnancy but had given birth at full term. Knowing this, I wanted to believe that the same would happen to me. Nevertheless I couldn't stop worrying and each time I rang the doctor I asked what would happen if I did indeed miscarry. Each time I was told that as I was only two months pregnant, a miscarriage would be just like a heavy period with the same kind of slight stomach cramps. Each time, though, it was stressed that I shouldn't worry until I felt any pain, only then would a miscarriage be inevitable.

I spent the next two days in bed doing nothing but worry. Then, early on Tuesday morning I was awakened by severe pains in my stomach and back. I cried and cried as, over the next two hours, a pattern of contractions built up. The pains built up and died away just like the descriptions of labour I had been reading. The pain was intense and nothing like a period. At the same time I was too upset to be frightened by what was happening. After the pains died away there was still no sign of bleeding. When the surgery opened I rang my doctor. Yet again I was treated over the phone. He suspected that the pain without bleeding could mean an ectopic pregnancy and asked me to get dressed and go down to the hospital for examination.

As I washed and got dressed I suddenly felt a rush of movement inside. A flood of foul-smelling blood came out and with it what looked like the sac which would have held my child. I screamed and screamed from shock and M [female friend] came running to help me. M cleared up while I lay in bed once again. I was stunned by what had happened, by the sight of the sac and the blood. The feeling of it coming out was vivid and I felt as though I had given birth instead of seeing the end of my child.

Carla's Story

Carla lost her baby at 12 weeks.

I didn't know how to think about it. I didn't know what labels to put on it or what names to give it. I had a non-viable pregnancy. My baby died after three months in the womb. I had an overripe egg. I was too old. I was too anxious. I was too happy. I had a simple medical procedure and went on with life, back at work the next day. I forestalled a miscarriage by having a D and C, on the doctor's assurance that nothing inside my womb was still alive.

I had not thought about miscarriage at all. No one in my family had miscarried. I married late, at 41, and became pregnant the first month we ceased to try to prevent it. So easy, it had to be right. It was planned, slotted into a very full, very busy life. My husband and I both worked at full-time jobs while attending law school at night. I had a position as an attorney lined up for the fall. When I became pregnant in December, it was obvious that I could just delay my start with the firm for a few months; the baby would be born two months after I took the bar exam, in September; I would have a little time to be a full-time mother, and go to work in January.

My first marriage was childless. My husband has a daughter by his first wife, my step-daughter and the joy of my life. I was light-headed with happiness when I got pregnant. My husband was scared, but sent me flowers and got quite optimistic about it, though he had fiercely resisted the whole idea of a second family when we first met. For me, it was a prerequisite of our being together, he and I, that he understand that I wanted a family more than anything. We fought about it. I won.

Despite the lightness and happiness and confidence in the ease of getting pregnant, there was fear. Fear that at my age, I would produce a monster. Fear that my body would not tolerate the pregnancy, although I had been pronounced in perfect health. Fear of genetic disorders. Fear of physical pain.

My doctor suggested that I not wait four months to do amniocentesis, but instead we have a new test done called 'chorionic villus sampling'. The idea of the test is that you get almost all the same information as from amnio, but at nine weeks instead of at 16. Since the exact age of the foetus is critical for this test, it is preceded by an early ultrasound. I scheduled the ultrasound, and my husband arranged to meet me at the hospital since we were to have some genetic counselling at the same time.

The ultrasound showed a problem. They couldn't find something they were looking for. We were instructed to wait two weeks, and then come back and do it again. Maybe we had miscounted.

The impact of that neutral bit of information was stunning. I had been floating along, feeling tired and ecstatic about being pregnant and having swollen breasts and a precious secret. I squirmed with a sore back in the hard plastic bucket seats at law school, barely able to keep my eyes open to read my assignments after nine at night, but I went to work knowing that there was a good reason for the discomfort, that I could manage it, that I would be a mother. Suddenly, I felt fat and afraid, old and incompetent.

The two-week wait was the hardest wait of my life. I had told no one at work that I was pregnant (You're 42 and you're *what*? You want to be a big-time attorney and you're *what*?), so I couldn't look for support there. My husband refused to deal with the possibility that in two weeks I would have a D and C instead of having a baby in six months. He was not only no support, he chastised me for worrying about it, for no longer being joyful. I hated him; we hated each other for the whole two weeks. For myself, I still felt physically pregnant. I had all the same symptoms. I had no pain. I wasn't bleeding or cramping. How could anything be wrong?

Well, in two weeks I went through the ultrasound again, this time without my husband. I didn't want him there. A woman friend came with me, and heard with me that whatever had been inside me was dead, not growing. It was easier to hear this than to wait out the previous two weeks.

The medical ending was simple: a day surgery D and C, back to work the following day, no physical ill effects. My husband and I became friends again. He wants to try again now, to have a child with me. The emotional effect, for me, is still not over. I lost not only one three-month foetus, but the confidence that I could, physically and/or emotionally, have a child. I write this eight months after the miscarriage. I have not had the courage to try again.

Well, first I was told to wait three or four months. So that covered the spring. And then I had to take the bar exams, high stress levels, not a good time to become pregnant. And now I have started my new job in a large, high-powered law firm, the kind of firm that had no women at all as attorneys 12 years ago, and now has just a few and most of them without children. And I do not have the courage – I would like to say 'yes' – to go through it all again. To be that tired, and that excited, and that scared, and that miserable and rejected by my spouse for the misery. And that secretive. And also, that old. Since I turned 40, my body is changing, getting heavier no matter how many miles I run or bicycle or ski.

Somewhere in the back of my mind I think I always had the confidence that when the time was right, I could have a child. That it failed, just that once, doesn't seem to be objectively to make a difference – after all, 20 per cent of all pregnancies end in miscarriage, I'm told. But it made a difference for me. I lost the confidence that it would be okay. I hope it comes back soon.

Helen's Story

Helen was operated on for an ectopic pregnancy at the end of the first trimester. There was a possibility of a twin conception.

When I read what I wrote in hospital, it all came back. There were about 35 or 40 of us in the gynae ward at a large London hospital. We had some gynaecological problems, or we were women who had something else wrong with us and this was the convenient place. Cyst, laparoscopy, laparotomy, hysterectomy, miscarriage, ectopic, cancer of the breast, liver, ovary, cervix, terrible peeling skin disease; also 'the exploratory' and 'the test'. It is a surgical ward. Some of us had pieces cut out or sucked out, and others, admitted for the aptly named 'test', have just learned that they have failed and will die. The women who have just learned that their baby is all right or they *don't* have cancer after all are somewhere else, perhaps already home. Certainly not here.

I am in for an ectopic pregnancy; the foetus has been growing in the fallopian tube, not the womb. In the ward we are all experts in our own misfortune, or we learn fast. There is apparently no way to save an ectopic baby. Left untreated, the tube would eventually burst, causing severe haemorrhaging and death, if one were not already in hospital or very close indeed. Even an 'early' ectopic is a serious business, with a potential for peritonitis and a certainty of nasty pain.

My surgeon found me an object of interest, as he explained: an ectopic occurs about once every 280–300 pregnancies in Britain, though they happen more frequently in tropical countries such as Jamaica (about one in 30). Often they are misdiagnosed as miscarriages, at least initially. The likelihood of an ectopic does not increase with age, and previous childbearing does not guarantee immunity. My surgeon proceeded methodically, first removing the contents of my womb via the vagina. Then, finding more of what he euphemistically called 'products of conception' than he had expected, he made a small incision and did a laparoscopy which revealed the pregnancy in the tube. He then made a larger incision across my lower abdomen (like a Caesarian, I was told, only longer) and removed the foetus and what remained of the tube. The sum total of 'products' made him think that I might have actually lost twins, possibly one in the womb and another in the tube; that would have made me one in 30,000! I always knew I was special. He was sending off material to be tested but I didn't want to know the result.

The gynae ward is a floating world. While we are inside, there is no other world. Each of us has two possessions, our illness and our story. It is those of us between 30 and 50, whatever our social background, who tend to tell our stories. Those younger and older may describe their condition, but rarely their life. Some say nothing, but weep. There is a lot of crying. Even the stories are incomplete, because they always end in the ward.

The ward itself is the way our bodies seem to us. It functions, but just barely, at the acute centre. All around, everything is falling apart. Every weekend they run out of linen; if your bed is bloodied, and some are, tough luck. No paper towels in the loo – very sanitary, that – and the roll of paper towelling at the nurses' sink, strictly monitored, runs out every mid-afternoon. Did they also run out of loo paper? I remember asking for some from home. Peeling paint, dirt on the non-opening windows, no working pay phones. And the savings from this must have been minimal.

I got into the ward through love and fate. When Graham and I married, I was already over 40 and had two children. He had none. So we would have one, one that would be 'ours', not 'hers', and lo and behold, five months after our marriage I became pregnant. I felt proud of my fertility and proud of what felt like a homage to our love. In between came lurches of fear about bringing up children virtually until I would be 60, fear about money, career, creativity, strength. But it felt like fate: so be it.

Then, near the end of the third month, things began to go wrong. Some bleeding, a tight, heavy feeling in the abdomen that gradually became pain, and a whitish, almost elastic discharge. Pregnancy test positive, another pregnancy test positive, down to the hospital for an internal: 'Looks like a pregnant uterus to me.' Referral to ultrasound, where for the first time in my life I see the image of my own womb, not like a triangle but like a lyre, its walls thick as pillars. Beautiful and strong. No baby visible. Sometimes the machine does miss the baby, but it's probably a miscarriage in process, I am told, or sometimes there can be false positive tests with women nearing menopause, hormonal signals go off, etc. Some other discussion about middle-aged hormones. My morale drops.

At this point I think there was another positive test. All this time I am in no doubt that what is happening is not a miscarriage and I am still pregnant, but I keep being shuttled back and forth. My GP has begun to suspect an ectopic, and he remarks that before the cuts someone like me would have been taken into hospital just to be sure. And another week passes; I feel I am being troublesome by not having a miscarriage and going away. Meanwhile the pain has become steady and I feel heavy, waxen, dull.

More to the point, I am making mistakes. Because I want the baby to be all right, I try to go on with life as usual, going to work, exhausting myself. On Sunday I feel terrible but I am doggedly getting ready to go up to the university the next morning. Graham says, 'You're staying here and seeing the doctor.' 'Look,' I say in the superior accents of duty, 'my work isn't going to go away, anything I don't do this week, I'm only going to have to make up the following week.' And so on. We quarrel. I have been told that I am rather a workaholic, but what I didn't know was that on that Sunday I was arguing for my right to literally work myself to death. I was ill, three days away from an emergency operation, but to me, everybody was simply getting in my way. So here, at least, is a lesson: When you are seriously ill – especially if you don't want to be – your judgement is off. Graham was right, I was wrong.

On Monday we phoned the doctor who, I believe, had just had back another positive test. He said he felt I was in danger and he had a friend at the hospital who could get me in through emergency if I went in when he was on duty. This is what we did. But what if he hadn't had 'connections'? During admission, another internal, this time electrifyingly painful when he probed on the right side. Next day, in hospital, another unsucccessful scan. By now the pressure on my abdomen makes me cry. Next day they do a foolproof pregnancy test, but the hospital no longer does this in their own lab, so it has to be sent over to Hammersmith. I hear the houseman arguing on the phone about the cost of the taxi to take it over. Meanwhile I feel much worse, the discharge smells, and a decision is made to operate before the results of this last test come back.

When I returned from hospital 11 days after the operation, I was still terribly weak. I couldn't sit up or lie on my stomach. My family bustled about but my thoughts were on death. No baby, and my sense of bodily integrity, my sense of my body as something whole and healthy, gone too. The depression came in waves, maybe the work of my hormones, maybe that and my thoughts and post-operative shock. Never let anyone tell you that a Caesarian, with full anaesthetic, has about the same effect on the body as normal childbirth! Any abdominal operation is major surgery.

Convalescent weakness is unlike ordinary weakness in that effort gets you nowhere. The reserve strength isn't there. I went back to work after seven weeks, exactly as recommended, but I wasn't really ready for it. I would get into bed after work and all weekend. I felt low and I walked around hunched over. My job seemed unreal. Food looked weird, who'd want the stuff? My body felt like a potato on sticks. The persistence of this aftermath took me totally by surprise. It was six months before I found myself feeling energetic and a year before I was feeling the same about myself.

Yet I do not actually feel the same. The straight, dark scar ('Excellent work', said my GP) remains as a sardonic smile reminding me that you don't always get what you want. I look at it less now, but its message is the same. The day after my operation, the surgeon stopped by my bed, discussed his 'twins' theory, and chatted on about how my chances of another pregnancy were still pretty good, perhaps 60 per cent.[1] He had left the ovary, and, who knows, there had even been cases of pregnancies out of the womb or of eggs migrating in the abdomen. What is the cultural means of transmission of the medical half-lie? Do they pick it up as interns from consultants who have a particularly low view of patients' intelligence? As I learned later, the true percentage is about 40 per cent.[1] While he spoke I felt a rush of irrational hatred for him. Who was this man, who the hell was he to have had his hands inside me, why didn't he check if what was in my womb was alive? But I didn't say a word. He had done a good job on the operation itself and at least I had been able to speak to him before; using the jargon, I had said, please be conservative, leave as much as you can. I assume he did.

This crisis has set the shape for much of my life since. Graham and the children have formed a much closer friendship and he says this is enough for him, he doesn't feel such an urgent need for a child of his own. The hospital offered us its in-vitro programme[2] to get round the one-tube problem, but we declined. I have been able to admit to myself that I want to use this time in my life for my work and for the relationships I already have. The convalescence forcibly brought home to me that my body has limits and that no one is helped if I push myself to my absolute physical edge with work. So I have been trying to do one thing at a time instead of feeling I should be doing everything all the time. I haven't noticed any decline in results.

Yet there has been a loss, and I am not sure I have quite finished mourning for it. One sign of this incomplete process is that I find it embarrassing to write about the pain or tears or depression, as if they were dirty or I was indulging myself by having them. So I have not quite gone through the entire healing process. I know why I'm writing about this, though. A private experience has mainly private consequences, but bearing witness to it takes it out of the silence in which so much women's experience has been buried. It makes it available so that at least we know the range of a woman's life. Although it only happened to me, to my body, it could have been the experience of any woman.

I've noticed, writing this, that I've sometimes called what was lost 'it' or 'them' or 'the baby' or 'the foetus' or myself. It was all these things. It wasn't yet a person, but it was a futurity, it meant life. There's a deep human instinct to seek meaning and value, even in a disaster as random as the weather. Every cloud has a silver lining, it's an ill wind that blows nobody good. For every drop of rain a flower grows. The old wisdom is right, but like all oracles it must not be taken literally. When I told myself that it was all for the best because it had brought us closer as a family, I felt worse than ever. Something has been lost, something gained, but they are different things. One doesn't sponge out the other. I think it's very important to let them be discrete and not to try to force, say, a living relationship or an art work into the space of a loss. The spirit resists it. Better to experience both and to honour life by not trying to make everything in it equivalent to something else.

There have been a few times – very few – when Graham has been angry about our family and something about not having a child comes out, and I feel desolate, and he apologises. Or we go to a barbecue, as we did yesterday, and there are twins in a pram who are the right age and I won't look in the pram and I feel like a stickwoman for the rest of the day, and Graham says, 'Ours would have been the same age,' because he's been thinking the same thing.

So we do still have some impulse towards a child. We did make a decision not to try again, but (like all big decisions?) it trails behind it a wake of alternatives. We have resolved to use this time for our creativity, and we do use it. I think this is the right decision, but I wanted – in some way I still want – that baby.

Janet's Story

Janet miscarried her first baby at seven and a half weeks.

My miscarriage happened ten months ago. My body returned to its normal cycle of fertility quite soon. But my life, my relationships, my feelings, my emotions, my thoughts, my perceptions have not returned to my pre-pregnancy normality. They never will. I am a different person, one I sometimes don't recognise. For me the loss of my baby was a loss of innocence. And this is a quality which cannot be regained.

I was 32, had been in the relationship with my husband for nearly 14 years. We had become aware of issues about contraception and its implications for my body and our relationship. We had decided to practise a natural method and as a result had become very familiar with and responsive to all the information my body had to give. We knew the day when I ovulated and when there was no possibility of my becoming pregnant. We had done everything we wanted to do. We both liked children and felt that we could deal with making a decision about having a family of our own.

We consulted my menstrual charts, decided when we'd like a baby to be born, consulted our natural family planning teachers and friends, especially one who is an obstetrician; decided to try to conceive a boy (an arbitrary choice, but one which natural family planning makes more possible); charted and monitored my cycle with great care until the exact moment: Thursday, 29 January 1981. We were successful. We were expecting a baby. My charts showed it, and I knew it. We cancelled a holiday in South-east Asia because I could not have any vaccinations and decided to go to Japan for a month instead (no vaccinations, very clean, very safe, good hospitals – just in case). I remember saying, when we'd changed all our arrangements, 'After all this, it'd be just my luck to have a miscarriage.' But they were just words.

And so we went to our doctor, a man of infinite openness and understanding, close to the National Childbirth Trust, happy to accept the evidence of my charts. And so I was duly registered pregnant. No one knew except us, the GP and one close friend, also, by chance, a doctor. I had no pregnancy test, it was not necessary. My parents came to stay, also by chance, and we told them the news.

Then, on Friday, 6 March I was sick and faint and had pains in my stomach for an hour or two and my mother fell into her old role of looking after me through it. My husband felt inadequate and we all knew what we were thinking but none of us said. The next day we went out for a trip and I had pains in my stomach. The pictures of me then show it, but not to others, who just say I looked pretty. On Sunday my parents left. At lunchtime on Monday I started bleeding and from one o'clock until five thirty p.m. I walked from mirror to mirror, crying and wailing and talking to myself 'No it can't be true. Yes it is. It isn't necessarily. Don't panic. Please come home R [husband]. Please, somebody phone me. Who can I talk to? Don't be silly. I must see if it's stopped yet. Mummy bled when she expecting me.' On and on, round and round, from bedroom to bathroom to toilet to window to hallway and back again. It was the beginning of knowing that I really cared, that I was involved with this little person inside me, that I could feel and experience depths that I didn't know about. At the age of 32 years and two months, after a relationship of 13 and a half years, at the first time of trying, I had conceived a child. A child, not a foetus, a child. Our first child. I just hadn't realised. Up until I saw the blood and felt the threat of loss, it had all seemed like an organisational problem.

At five thirty my husband came home. I told him that I was bleeding and I cried, and he put his arms around me as though *I* needed comforting. He didn't seem to see it like I did. He didn't seem to realise the significance of what I was saying. I was unable to explain because the experience itself was all I could cope with, I could not also interpret it. We were unprepared for grief and fear and so R, after a little while, began to tell me of some important events of his day and inside I was screaming, 'But I'm bleeding! Don't you understand? I'm bleeding!' And I thought he would hear me, and know what to do. But he didn't. At that point I began to feel that I was alone in this. We had always been together. We had believed that pregnancy, labour, delivery was *our* experience, not just mine. But the physical experience could not be shared, and it is the physical experience that reminds you, every minute, every second. All the time, *all* the time. There is nothing else worth talking or thinking about. It doesn't leave you alone. 'Pure' feelings of grief and fear became contaminated with 'nasty' feelings of resentment and anger and frustration in being unable to communicate, and disappointment that, after all, I did not have the unity I thought I had.

Every morning the bleeding stopped and every afternoon it

started and on the Wednesday we went back to our doctor. He felt, palpated, and prodded and questioned that I had ever been pregnant at all: 'You told me you were pregnant and I believed you.' And I, knowing that I had been pregnant, started to doubt myself and my knowledge of my body. I felt concerned for the doctor, that he felt he had made a mistake, and it was my fault. You are very willing to believe that everything is your fault. R kept saying, 'You *were* pregnant.' The doctor sent off for a pregnancy test and so did our best friend. On Thursday he telephoned to say that the results were negative, but that it was remotely possible that this was wrong. But I was glad that a friend had told me. On Friday we went back to the GP who also said, 'It's negative,' and wanted to know if I'd lost 'any bits of meat'. No, I hadn't lost any bits of meat. And he was very good, and told me that I didn't have to put a brave face on it. He helped to justify my feelings. Half way through our talk with him, we realised that friends were coming to dinner, so R went and wrote a note to them and came back. The GP phoned the hospital because I had not lost any bits of meat and he didn't know whether I'd ever been pregnant. I was afraid that the whole episode had just been hysteria, and he was thinking 'neurotic woman'.

We went home and retrieved our friends. The woman said not a word about it and her man said, 'Sorry about the trouble.' We had dinner, like nothing was wrong, and I had a little baby inside me who could be dead or alive. I seemed to be the only one who gave it a second thought.

The next day, Saturday morning, we went to the teaching hospital where the obstetrics registrar saw us. I had been a lecturer at this medical school. I knew the registrar. He was as good as his 'medical model' training would allow him to be. He was very good. He talked to us for a long time, answered our questions, told us what he was thinking. He said it could be due to anything: 'No, it's not possible to find out why, but if it happens again we'll worry and it if happens a third time, we'll investigate. It's a common occurrence.' Common to him, but not to me.

So, since we weren't sure about what was going on inside me, he suggested an ultrasound scan, which gives a little TV picture of the uterus and its contents. This was arranged and we went to the ultra-sound machines and he went to his technical work. The screen showed that I was or had been pregnant. He measured it all on the screen and worked it all out, how old the foetus was: seven and a half weeks. He explained it all and was marvellously clear.

And I had seen my baby. I had known that I was pregnant, and I had doubted it, doubted me, doubted this little baby's existence because some forms of knowledge are seen as more valid than others.

And I had been shown my baby, still inside me. S/he had been measured and given an age. And I had shown detached interest in the wonders of technology. And it was the depth of my despair, the loudest of my silent screaming, the most desolate loneliness. All inadmissable. And if this baby had died, it had not also left me. 'But we cannot be absolutely certain that it is not alive. So let's leave it for a while, see what happens, look again.' Six days of not knowing whether I was carrying life or death inside me. And it would not be determined for five more days. And in those days we went to dinner with friends, a colleague of R's arrived from Sweden to stay with us for three months, I had my varicose veins injected at that same hospital, we went to a film. And all the time wondering if I'm saying out loud, 'I'm having a miscarriage. Can you see this dead baby inside me?' And resentment and anger and loneliness and despair. And remembering that our close friend the doctor had once suggested that I was not in any physical state to have babies because I did not eat enough. My fault. And my father saying that I should not have lifted that sewing machine. My fault. And the obstetrician saying that nothing I did or didn't do would have caused this. Not my fault. But even so, it was my body that produced it. And your life goes on, or the events of it do, and all the time this terrible thing is happening to you.

On the Thursday at five o'clock we went back to the hospital and the ultrasound and the TV pictures and the calculations. The baby was smaller than before. Definitely dead, and had been so for some time. It wasn't such a shock. I'd seen the pictures before. I knew what to expect. I discussed it all so sensibly. The obstetrician had forgotten all about involving my husband, who had to search all the rooms to find us. I thought that I could be 'sensible' about it all. Of course, we couldn't let the dead foetus come out of its own accord, especially since it might happen in Japan where we were going in ten days' time. So a D and C was definitely indicated. The obstetrician explained it, drew the instruments, did everything he could. He said that I might as well have it done at eight p.m., it being six p.m. now. I'd not eaten anything, just in case. And so it was. I wanted to say, 'Keep the baby, don't throw it down the sluice. I want to see it.' I didn't dare in case he thought I was mad and morbid and dwelling on things and wallowing in it all instead of pulling myself together. I had my D and C, a 'scrape', and they scraped my baby out and made me clean and hygienic again and told me not to get pregnant again for a couple of months because of a higher incidence of foetal abnormalities straight after a miscarriage. The next morning I went home. No longer pregnant. No longer having a miscarriage. But it's not over then, it's only just beginning. Now comes the emotional wreckage.

Penny's Poem

Miscarriage

Three times then
Seeping loss
And with each seeping
A child becoming nothing
An empty hollow pain
A flushing away –
Then grief.
The thwarted readiness
The loneliness
And creeping doubt to follow
Sure as guilt.
The third time I remembered:
I read somewhere
About some Indians
Who went through this
Some peaceful camping women in America
They lost their babies
All of them
I don't recall the place now
But they tested bombs near there.

Who will answer us then?
Those of you who reassure
Those of you who permit
Will you tell us
That your safe low level radiation
Is low enough, safe enough,
For new formed beings
Clinging to the vine
Trying to be born?
Do you take
Some measure of care?
And how then

Would we know?
On whose information
Should we base our choices
For the unborn?
Or are they, in some strange way,
As wise as their ancestors,
Those Indians
Who do not come.

Penny Henrion

Part Two:
Medical Viewpoints

Introduction:
Understanding What
Happened and Why

Mary Anne Speakman

Nearly all the women contacted during the research for this book voiced the need to know more about why miscarriages and/or ectopic pregnancies happen and bewailed the lack of such information in medical handbooks and even women's health books. Recently, this omission has been rectified, to some extent, by the publication of a few books on miscarriage, which, together with this book, will add to the body of knowledge accessible to women who wish to find out more about their pregnancy loss. If reading these chapters sparks anything off in your mind that is not dealt with here, then the first person to consult would probably be your GP. Ask for a referral to the consultant at your local hospital or further afield if you feel this would help. If you're not satisfied, contact your local Community Health Council for advice. Hopefully, you will receive a sympathetic hearing, especially if you go in prepared to explain your need for help in an assertive but not aggressive manner. It is worth remembering, too, that you can choose a different GP for maternity care (as opposed to general health care) in a subsequent pregnancy.

Usually, the miscarriage or ectopic pregnancy leads to quite a flurry of activity on the part of doctors and nurses: examinations, taking your medical history, giving injections, preparing for the operating theatre. Exactly what did happen to you may be rather vague and it is not until afterwards that you wonder why some medical procedure or test was carried out. Understanding your GP's actions and what happened to you at the hospital can be an important part of understanding your loss – sorting out a few details, clarifying a few points, laying a few ghosts to rest. This is why information on the roles of the GP and hospital doctor and the various procedures involved in caring for a woman who is miscarrying or having an ectopic pregnancy is included in this book.

The need to know why miscarriages and ectopic pregnancies occur is a real one for many women and quite detailed information is provided here. However, as has been pointed out, the reasons why a great many miscarriages occur are just not known and yours may be one of the many miscarriages with no obvious cause. This can be hard to accept; if there is a reason for something, it's often easier to come to terms with it and to do something to prevent it happening again. At the very least, the information given here may help to eliminate some possibilities and, if you are hoping to conceive again, the information on genetic counselling and ante-natal diagnostic techniques will be of value. The state of medical knowledge and related technology is constantly changing – this section has been updated several times during the preparation of this book – so it is possible that in the future further reasons for miscarriage and ectopic pregnancy will become known and treatments devised to prevent their recurrence.

In Part Three questions are raised as to the way the usual medical model circumscribes the explanations given, the words used, the treatments and care received during women's experience of miscarriage or ectopic pregnancy. For example, the medical model can suggest causes of miscarriage but does not have adequate resources to show how bodies and emotions interact. When suggesting causes on an objective level, it is important not to lose sight of women's subjective understanding of what is going on inside their bodies and souls.

Whilst recognising the need to include as much detailed and honest medical information as possible, we (as editors) were, therefore, concerned not to put it above the other issues that have become, over the course of coming to terms with our own losses and in the writing of this book, at least as important as why we had a miscarriage or ectopic pregnancy, if not more so. How women's experience in hospital is related to perceptions of women as potential mothers is one such issue. Both Gill Yudkin and Fran Reader, as the medical practitioners who have written this part of the book, were highly aware of the inadequacy of the medical model and the insensitive practices that could result. The procedures and treatments they describe will be fairly common to all GP surgeries and hospitals, but the woman-centred context proposed to encompass such care represents an ideal. Sadly, few women have as yet experienced this type of caring. However, by removing the mystique from medical knowledge, at least women can come to understand their experience better and attempt to engage in informed discussion with their doctors if they wish.

From Home to Hospital and Back

Gill Yudkin

The Role of the GP

The traditional family doctor is (or can be) the one person in a woman's life who may know her from her birth to her death. She or he may be involved in many of this woman's life events, both happy and sad. The doctor may attend her bedside when she is ill, comfort her when others close to her are ill or die, rejoice with her as she establishes a new relationship with a partner or starts a new job, care for her through pregnancy and confinement or care for her and comfort her when she suffers pre-term loss of pregnancy.

This rewarding aspect of general practice, the continuity of care, is less common today, partly because patients move around so much, not just within their town or city, but around the country, and partly because of how general practice is now organised. The majority of doctors work in partnerships or large groups. Many do not do their own night calls but employ a deputising service; those who do their own out of hours calls will probably have a rota for this work. This means that even if a woman has been registered with a particular GP all her life, she will not necessarily have access to that doctor during a crisis.

Many women nowadays confirm their own pregnancies very early, using the new highly sensitive immunological tests which are readily available at chemist shops. A pregnancy can be confirmed even before the first period is missed, so what might in the past have been called a late period is now diagnosed as an early miscarriage, possibly increasing the emotional burden on some women.

Pregnancy is an exciting time and many women are keen to get antenatal care under way as soon as possible and make their first visit to the GP as early as five or six weeks gestation. This can be a time for general advice about pregnancy and a reminder of the advantage of taking folic acid supplements if they haven't already begun. It is also a time for reinforcing advice about reducing alcohol and cigarette consumption, but referral to a hospital antenatal clinic is not usually made until about ten weeks.

Most antenatal care is shared between the GP and the local hospital obstetric unit. However, increasingly, community midwives are taking over, particularly from the hospital side, with varying success as far as cooperation from the GPs is concerned. As an example of the variation in service available, I work in a district which is divided down the middle. On one side of the main road which divides our practice area, women have the advantage of a superb community midwife-led programme. There are two midwives based at the local teaching hospital unit who do all the antental books at home, conduct a weekly antenatal clinic with the GPs at our health centre and do either domino deliveries in the community suite at the hospital or home confinements. Communication between the GPs and midwives is extremely good, thus benefiting the patients. On the other side of the main road, however, the system is much less satisfactory with more remote midwives, no home booking and much less effective communication all round. There are different models of care all over the city and indeed the country. If communication with the midwives is good, and the unhappy event of a pre-term loss occurs, the midwife may be the main support for the woman.

However, it is to be hoped that the family doctor will be involved as early as possible in the crisis and available for follow-up care. Before the Second World War it was not uncommon for a woman to have several miscarriages and she would rarely have a contact with any doctor at all, especially a hospital doctor. Nowadays, a large majority of women suffering a miscarriage will be admitted to hospital, but their stays will be brief. Even with an ectopic pregnancy, the hospital stay will rarely be for more than one week.

Nevertheless, much of the experience of a woman suffering pre-term loss of pregnancy will focus on the hospital experience. The hospital doctors, in their very brief contact with the woman, shape the lasting impression she carries away with her about the care she had during her sad experience. The hospital doctor does not then have the benefit or the problems of the long-term follow up.

The GP, however, is there to stay, although, of course, if a patient has a bad experience of care from the GP she may try to change her doctor. The family doctor, unlike the hospital doctor, has more opportunity to learn from each patient. One realises how very different are the experiences of each individual and how reactions are dependent on so many different factors – physical, social and emotional.

It would be easy to write a scenario for a straightforward

miscarriage but it does not really happen like that. Just as every person is unique, so is every pregnancy and so is every miscarriage. There are no set rules; each miscarriage is managed according to its own special circumstances, according to the person and her situation and according to the personality and sensitivities of the medical personnel involved. We can look back on each miscarriage and criticise its handling – not just by the doctor but by the woman too. It can be helpful to criticise but if criticism turns to blame it can become harmful. We can learn by mistakes but we grow bitter from blame.

The GP becomes involved in a miscarriage in many different situations and at varying stages. The pregnancy may not yet have been confirmed, or if it has been confirmed, the GP may not know about it. The pregnancy may have been planned but, even if not planned, it may be a wanted pregnancy. Indeed, termination may have been considered and rejected by the patient or wanted by the patient and refused by the doctor – or a termination may already have been arranged but the date of the operation not yet reached.

The miscarriage may occur in a first pregnancy or a later pregnancy. It may be after previous miscarriages and the patient may have already had a child. When miscarrying, the knowledge that she is capable of producing a live child is of great importance to the woman. A miscarriage is often felt as a failure. The loss could be in early pregnancy before the woman felt 'really pregnant' or it could be later, when movements had already been sensed and the reality of a child inside her had become apparent. She may already have had a scan and actually seen her baby. Some scan departments make a photograph of the screen for the parents to take away. This photograph could be very helpful in the grieving process.

Each set of circumstances puts a miscarriage in a different context. To the GP, a miscarriage is a commonplace occurrence, almost a normal 'life event', but to the patient it may be the most traumatic episode in her life, with far reaching and devastating consequences. She may never feel the same person again.

Diagnosing Miscarriage

The GP's involvement in a miscarriage is different from and more prolonged than the hospital doctor's. Initially, there is a diagnosis. Is this a miscarriage or not, given that bleeding in early pregnancy is very common? A 'threatened miscarriage' (or 'abortion') is a term used to describe a situation where there has been some bleeding and perhaps a little pain, but the neck of the womb (the cervix of the uterus) stays tightly closed and the pregnancy is continuing. If the bleeding continues and the neck of the womb starts opening, this is an 'inevitable abortion' and the pregnancy inevitably ends. A 'complete abortion or miscarriage' is when everything empties out of the womb by itself, the neck of the womb closes again and there is no further bleeding. In practice, this rarely happens and the miscarriage is 'incomplete', with bleeding continuing and surgical intervention needed to help the womb to empty completely.

The terminology used by medical personnel may be quite distressing to the woman who is miscarrying. Abortion is the medical word used to describe the loss of a pregnancy before 24 weeks. This may be either a spontaneous abortion or miscarriage, or it may be a therapeutic abortion, a deliberate termination of pregnancy for medical or social reasons. There has come to be a stigma attached to the word abortion, which implies an induced termination of pregnancy. We must remember, however, that many, if not the majority, of women undergoing a therapeutic abortion may be as sad and distressed at their loss as women who are miscarrying may be.

With modern neonatal technology, some babies born before 28 weeks and even as early as 25 weeks gestation survive and do well. It is for this reason that the law controlling therapeutic abortions (termination of pregnancy) has recently been changed to permit the operation only up to 24 weeks, instead of 28 weeks as previously, except in exceptional circumstances. A stillbirth is a pregnancy loss from 24 weeks, when there is no sign of any breath having been taken.

Bleeding is usually the first sign of a miscarriage, but bleeding does not always indicate a miscarriage. It may be just a late period, especially if the pregnancy has not yet been confirmed or there are no other symptoms of pregnancy (such as excessive tiredness, frequent passing of urine, sore or full breasts, nausea).

If pregnancy has been confirmed but is not yet very far advanced – say less than ten weeks since the first day of the last normal period – then the bleeding could be just one of the many instances of insignificant bleeding in early pregnancy, the kind of slight bleeding that does not herald anything serious. However, it is a good thing to inform the doctor and ask for advice. The situation can often be clarified by an ultrasound scan.

In some units, even when most care is in the hands of midwives, an ultrasound scan is performed before any other tests or the initial examination. This is helpful to date a pregnancy and also to confirm viability. Sometimes the uterus is found to be smaller than would be expected from the date of the last period and there are no normal embryo parts seen. This is a missed abortion, where the embryo has died but the decidua and membranes have not been expelled. There may be no symptoms and the woman has no indication that her pregnancy is not progressing normally. However, she may lose all her symptoms of pregnancy, such as nausea and breast tenderness. In addition there may be a dull, low abdominal ache and brownish, waterly vaginal discharge. If left alone, it would eventually (maybe after another month) progress to an inevitable miscarriage with heavy bleeding and pain. However, there is a risk of infection superseding, or, even more rarely, a problem with the woman's blood clotting mechanisms, so an ERPC is usually recommended. This also avoids a harrowing wait for the woman who knows that her baby has died.

Not every episode of bleeding requires a home visit by the doctor or an examination. Advice may well be just to wait and see and to take things easy. However much the patient needs reassurance, the doctor may also choose not to visit if she or he is satisfied that nothing serious or dangerous is happening.

This is where the doctor's prior knowledge of the woman (as her GP) may be crucial. Reassuring someone over the telephone if one knows the patient well is a realistic possibility. Reassurance by a strange doctor or even by a message through a receptionist may be deemed quite unreassuring by the patient.

The seriousness of the situation will be judged on a description of the bleeding, whether it is just pinkish or brownish staining or the more serious frank red blood; whether it is just spotting or coming steadily (and it is a good idea to save any stained pads, clothes or towels, to give an estimate of blood loss); whether there is pain. Light spotting without pain usually settles. It may recur each month for a few months at the time of the expected period. It is probably a good idea to have a pregnancy test a few days after the bleeding has stopped, to make sure the pregnancy is continuing. If symptoms of pregnancy are still going on, that is a good sign that the pregnancy is still going on – symptoms stop very quickly after a miscarriage and even before the outward signs of pain and bleeding. So often, patients say that they were just beginning to feel 'better', to be less tired and nauseated. If the bleeding is heavy or if there is associated pain, there is rather more urgency and the GP should be called immediately. As has been mentioned, some GPs are more available than others, so in these circumstances, if the GP cannot be contacted at once it is wise to go straight to the casualty department of a hospital – by car if there is one readily available or by ambulance (by dialling 999) if not.

If the GP is available, an internal examination may be done to assess the state of the neck of the womb, or cervix. If this is open, then it means the miscarriage is 'inevitable' and the decision then is whether to wait and see if it all 'completes' on its own or whether the woman should be admitted to hospital for a D and C or ERPC.

The GP may not perform an internal examination, knowing that the management rarely hinges on this and that if the patient has to go to hospital, she will be subjected to probably more than one further vaginal examination once she is there. The decision to admit to hospital depends partly on the woman's general condition, for example whether she has lost a large amount of blood and may need a transfusion. Also, any bits which have been passed should, if possible, be saved so that it can be estimated whether or not there has been a complete miscarriage with everything coming away. Most gynaecologists feel that a D and C should be done if the pregnancy was more advanced than six weeks.

If the bleeding is only slight, the doctor may just tell the patient to rest. It is in fact debatable whether or not bed rest achieves anything. There is nothing that really will save a pregnancy that has started to miscarry, but there is enormous pressure, especially on the doctor, to do something, so the harmless procedure of bed rest may be prescribed. Clearly if there are other children around this may cause more anxiety than reassurance and may not be at all practicable. But if a woman is in this situation, she should take things gently and try not to exert herself with heavy work. Penetrative sex is also best avoided until the pregnancy is firmly established.

A later miscarriage, during the second trimester may be heralded by the breaking of the waters or ruptured membranes which surround the baby in the uterus. This will be either a trickle of clear fluid or a rush, as often happens in labour at term. A late miscarriage is much more like labour, with painful contractions and delivery of a foetus which looks very much like a fully developed baby. This can all be accompanied by quite severe loss of blood. An early miscarriage can also give rise to the labour-like contractions.

A more rare occurrence is a hydatidiform mole, where a foetus does not develop at all but there is proliferation of placental tissue. This is yet another cause of bleeding and the blood may be as in an 'ordinary' miscarrige or it may be like tiny grapes. In addition, the woman may feel very sick because of abnormally high hormone levels. If a hydatidiform mole is suspected, the woman should be admitted to hospital for an ultrasound scan and subsequent evacuation of her uterus.

Providing Care

Once a miscarriage is reality, much explanation is necessary, not just about the physiological process but about possible reasons. In most cases, we (the doctors) just do not know why it has happened and very often it is difficult for a woman to accept this. Indeed it may be difficult for the doctor to admit it.

It is very important to reassure the patient that she did not cause the miscarriage, for example, by too much work, exercise or sex, or by eating the wrong foods or taking simple medicines either prescribed or bought over the counter. Doctors here may get wrongly blamed too, for example, for doing a vaginal examination earlier in the pregnancy. A bereaved patient (as indeed a woman is after a miscarriage) may need someone or something to blame. It is hard for a doctor who has done what is medically correct to have to receive this blame, but it is easier to bear if she or he really understands the emotions of the patient. Explanations are often needed, too, for aspects of the medical care and hospital process. Good communication between the GP and the hospital is very important but, again, often lacking because a miscarriage for a gynaecologist is so 'trivial'. It is also important that the doctors are in communication with other members of the health-care team as, for example, a midwife or a health visitor may be planning her routine antenatal visit and may not know that her client has miscarried.

The decision whether or not to admit the woman to hospital depends not just on her clinical condition but on other factors like whether she is alone, whether she has a telephone, how far away the nearest hospital is in case admission is needed later in an emergency, whether the GP is going to continue to be available, or whether there will be a handover of care to another doctor, either a known member of the practice or a deputy doctor who will probably be a stranger. Usually, however, the woman is admitted to hospital if the bleeding is heavy, if there is severe pain or if the pregnancy has already gone on for more than 12 weeks since the first day of the last period.

Hospitals vary enormously in their handling of women with miscarriages. Unfortunately, still, in most cases, although a miscarriage can be an emergency, it is afforded low priority by hospital staff and even when a woman has been assessed as needing an ERPC, she will be left for many hours until the end of an operating list. Indeed, the decision to operate may not even be made until the day after admission because ultrasound scanning 'out of hours' is only done in severe clinical conditions. The overnight wait may then be in an emergency ward with not just a variety of medical and surgical cases but sometimes in a mixed-sex ward. Although the GP cannot change things at the time, she or he can help by forewarning her of some of the possible problems. In the longer term, the GP can try to exert pressure on local 'provider units' (as our hospitals have come to be called!) to be more user-friendly. The GP must try always to be the patient's advocate but can also encourage patients to make official complaints if bad standards of care are encountered.

If a woman is pregnant and bleeding and if there is any doubt, then a doctor should be called even though in many cases not much more will be done than being told to rest and wait and see. The doctor needs more information than just physical details in order to assess the need for reassurance, or visiting or follow-up calls. The emotional significance of a pregnancy or a miscarriage may not be immediately apparent to a GP, especially if she or he is not the woman's own personal doctor. Whether the GP is or is not, however, much depends on whether the doctor makes it clear that it is permissible to be upset about losing a baby pre-term, whether the doctor appears sympathetic and empathetic enough to allow the woman to express her fear, grief, anxiety.

Late miscarriages are usually even more upsetting than early ones because the pregnancy has become a baby which is alive and moving in the womb. The woman who might have been ambivalent or disbelieving of her condition very early in pregnancy will very likely have started to relate to her unborn child. Late miscarriages often happen in hospital because of the more severe symptoms of blood loss and labour pain. Terminology here may be used insensitively – it is unfortunate if doctors and nurses talk about 'products of conception' when what they are referring to is the woman's baby with its placenta and membranes. The GP is less often involved at the time so it is especially important that the hospital contacts the GP as soon as possible. The health visitor and community midwife are even more likely to have been involved at this stage of the pregnancy and so they, too, should be alerted in order to avoid embarrassing and distressing encounters.

Ectopic Pregnancy

Ectopic pregnancy, or a pregnancy developing in the fallopian tube, requires much the same support but it is more dramatic and more traumatic, both in gynaecological terms and emotionally, than a miscarriage. It is a more difficult diagnosis to make, but failure to make the diagnosis may put the woman's life at risk. An ectopic pregnancy is a medical emergency and the patient should be admitted to hospital even if it is just suspected. Erring on the safe side in this way may put a woman through unnecessary anxiety and technical intervention, but must be balanced against the potential disaster of a missed diagnosis.

The early symptoms are brownish staining or slight blood loss fairly soon after a missed period – often before a pregnancy test has been performed. The bleeding is usually accompanied by pain on one side or the other low down in the abdomen. If the diagnosis is missed, the foetus grows in the tube until it is so big that the tube bursts, resulting in severe abdominal pain and often collapse of the patient due to blood loss into the peritoneal cavity (the inside of the abdomen). This can be precipitated by a vaginal examination so if the diagnosis is suspected it is far safer to refer the woman to hospital for a laparoscopy.

Explanations by the doctors involved are particularly important here, especially as the hospital doctors are liable to get carried away with the excitement of acute surgery. This is indeed 'Emergency Ward 10' stuff for the doctors but this will most certainly not be appreciated by the poor patient who is losing not just a pregnancy, a foetus, a baby, but part of her future childbearing apparatus. It almost always means the removal of the fallopian tube where the pregnancy is occurring. She needs reassurance, too, that the rest of this 'apparatus' is functional and healthy. The doctor must also remember that if it happens again, unlike with a miscarriage, she will not have another chance. She will also have undergone a frightening and painful experience.

Giving Advice and Emotional Support

Women react differently to having a miscarriage or an ectopic pregnancy. The GP must be sensitive but not so emotional that she or he allows the inappropriate guilt of the patient to be transferred to the doctor. The GP is the family doctor. The miscarriage or ectopic pregnancy might have been a member of the family. The medical condition will be cleared up quickly, the emotion surrounding it will not. There may be repercussions for some time to come.

Alison was 18 when she had a 'complete' miscarriage at home at seven weeks of pregnancy. She was unmarried but she and her boyfriend thought it would be fine to have a baby. A month after the miscarriage she came to the surgery to start the pill as she realised it was not an ideal time for the two of them to start a family after all (they were both unemployed and both still living with their respective parents). A month later, Alison came to see me again saying she was depressed and tearful and kept flying off the handle at people at home. She was very surprised when I made the link with her recent miscarriage. We talked for some time and she later failed to keep the appointment I offered her two weeks later. Two months later, however, she came for her repeat pill prescription and reported that she felt much better.

Sometimes the immediate response to a miscarriage is easily understandable. Diana is a secretary, aged 18. She was a bit irregular in her use of her diaphragm, having taken herself off the pill. She became pregnant, was upset about it and was referred for a termination. Ten days later, before her appointment for the termination, she had a miscarriage and had to be admitted to hospital for a D and C. Afterwards, she was very matter of fact about what had happened. Relief was her main emotion.

If, however, Diana had decided not to go ahead with the termination after all but to continue with her pregnancy, she might very well have felt very guilty after miscarrying. The fact that she had considered termination might have been blamed by her as the cause of the miscarriage – it might have been seen by some as retribution for her destructive thoughts.

At other times, the doctor may feel that the woman is excessively anxious, but when all the circumstances are known anxiety is indeed understandable. Jenny, a physiotherapist and mother of a two-year-old daughter, was very anxious about a little brown staining at six weeks because she was planning to go to India to work with her husband and had planned this pregnancy to make sure she had her baby in England before she left. A miscarriage at this stage would mean having to have a later baby delivered in circumstances she felt unsure of.

Catherine was very anxious about her slight bleeding because her husband was going to Germany that week and bed rest at home with an uncertain outcome without the support of her partner was a daunting, lonely and frightening prospect. Mary was 40 and a lesbian, and had conceived this, her first pregnancy, by AID (artificial insemination by donor). To conceive again was an increasingly remote possibility.

All of these women needed extra support and more home visits than were warranted on strictly medical grounds. By contrast there are women who seem to have much less emotional trauma than might be expected.

Annie, a very sanguine 23-year-old, had already suffered much trauma in her life. She had lost her mother and sister in a car crash, which had also left her very scarred. Happily married and with two children she had a complete miscarriage at eight weeks with no medical attention at all. Then in her fourth pregnancy, at ten weeks and having not yet reported her pregnancy, she arrived on foot at the surgery and ten minutes later fainted because of the severe blood loss she was suffering. She is now about to produce her third child, a year after that miscarriage.

Sylvia, married and working as a hotel receptionist, was a mystery to me. I first met her when she was 40 and just pregnant for the sixth time. She told me she was glad to be pregnant, having had two terminations and three miscarriages, none past ten weeks. I was anxious to refer her directly to a gynaecologist but she insisted on going on holiday the next week to Italy, where she miscarried yet again and had a D and C in Rome. Her insistence on having her holiday at such a vulnerable time implied that she might not have been particularly worried. Alternatively it might have been a sort of denial of her anxiety.

Women who have experienced loss may have significant anniversaries. One patient, whose live pre-term baby died after a few hours, felt particularly emotional one day and then realised that it had been the anniversary of the last menstrual period before her pregnancy. Another patient, Suzanne, married and in her thirties with a four-year-old son, miscarried while her sister was pregnant with her own first child. She was very sad and also very reassured by being told that the miscarriage was not because of her being so worried and concerned about her work. (I had explained to her that if worry could bring on a miscarriage then we would not need all the struggles and debates around the Abortion Act.) I felt she had 'got over' her miscarriage and was surprised that she became sad and low at the time of her expected delivery. Now, talking to other women who have miscarried, I realise this is very common even if the immediate grieving seems adequate.

Explanations are needed from the doctor and may, in fact, need to be repeated. In addition, emotional support may be sought, and indeed welcomed, not just by the woman, but by her partner and perhaps other members of her family. Equally, however, there may be a process of denial, a refusal to look at what has been a traumatic experience. The doctor is then in a difficult position, not knowing whether to seek out the patient or to try to make her examine her situation. Later, however, practical advice is needed, even though it may not be asked for, about contraception and the desirability of waiting a while before attempting to conceive again.

Reassurance about future pregnancies is often given although we can never promise that a miscarriage will not happen again. Nor can we give very much useful advice about how to reduce the likelihood of it happening again since we are unable to find the cause of most miscarriages. Because of this, we tend to refer for investigation only those women who have had two or even three consecutive miscarriages.

When another pregnancy does follow, the normal anxieties of any pregnant woman are exaggerated both up to, and especially around, the time of the preceding miscarriage. Extra support by the doctor is called for here and awareness of the particularly sensitive times. Early ultrasound scans are very helpful to show both the patient and her doctor that the pregnancy is proceeding normally.

I have described difficult circumstances in some women's lives which have had influences on their reactions to their miscarriages. To a lesser extent, circumstances in the life of the medical attendant may also colour the manner in which miscarriages are handled.

If the doctor is a woman, she may empathise totally with her patient, especially if she herself has had a miscarriage. If she does have this common background, however, she (the doctor) may actually be too emotional, hindering her clinical competence. If the doctor is a mother, while empathising with the patient, she may just feel relief that her pregnancy went to term. Many women doctors, though, have made a definite choice to follow their careers rather than to 'succumb' to their maternal feelings. This difficult choice may have given them a separateness and aloofness from the suffering of other women concerning maternity and its failure. And yet again there may be involuntary sterility in the doctor, giving rise to feelings of envy towards a patient who can at least conceive. It may be thought that a male doctor will not be caught up in such 'female' emotions, but of course his reactions will similarly depend upon his life situation and possibly his fertility and that of his partner. Whatever our personal situation, we must, as doctors, overcome these emotions and make ourselves not just available in practical terms but available and accessible emotionally to our patients.

Doctors have earned a bad reputation for being oppressive to women. Even feminist doctors are put into the same pigeon-hole as doctors in general and have to fight continually to be accepted as 'sisters'. The most fruitful way for all doctors to right their bad labels is by demonstrating that they are sensitive to others' feelings and that they use their skills not to oppress other women but to help, by sharing their skills and specialist knowledge and by demystifying the whole medical process.

The Reasons for Miscarriage and Ectopic Pregnancy

Fran Reader

Revised by Fran Reader and Kirsten Duckitt

Why Me?

Why do some pregnancies miscarry and some grow in the fallopian tube instead of the womb? Although nature is sometimes 'wonderful' in the field of reproduction, it can be a hit and miss affair. Consider the female turtle laying up to a thousand eggs into the warm Pacific island sands when only a few of the babies that hatch will eventually survive to be adult turtles. Consider human reproduction: sometimes a woman never becomes pregnant; sometimes a pregnancy ends after a few months. The problems may continue throughout pregnancy, for later on the baby may be born prematurely or deformed and not survive; or the baby may be born alive and healthy only to die in the early months of life.

Understanding 'why me?', and understanding the reasons why, are separate. It is impossible to understand 'why me?', but it can be helpful to know the medical reason for miscarriage. In many cases, however, the reason is not yet known; medical science cannot provide all the answers and offers only an incomplete picture of how our bodies and minds work. Let us look, though, at some of the various known causes of miscarriage or ectopic pregnancy to try to understand some of the reasons why.

Conception and the Development of the Baby

Every pregnancy begins with the fertilisation or union of an egg from the woman with a sperm from the man. The woman has two ovaries which contain many cells which can develop into a mature egg. Each month one of these cells matures and at a time about half way between periods, the egg is released. This is called ovulation. The egg passes into the nearby fallopian tube, where it can be

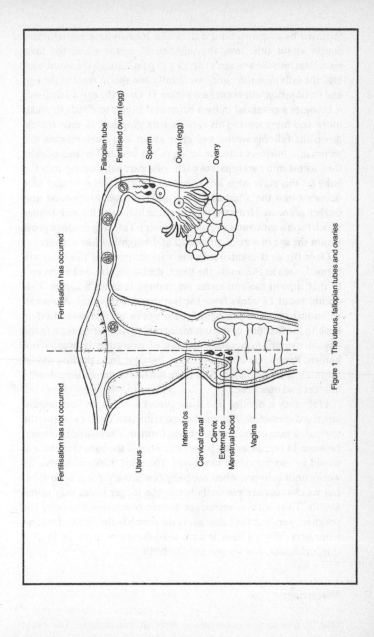

Figure 1   The uterus, fallopian tubes and ovaries

Labels:
- Fallopian tube
- Fertilised ovum (egg)
- Sperm
- Ovum (egg)
- Ovary
- Fertilisation has occurred
- Fertilisation has not occurred
- Uterus
- Internal os
- Cervical canal
- Cervix
- External os
- Menstrual blood
- Vagina

fertilised by a sperm. So if a man and woman have sexual intercourse about this time, the millions of sperm which the man ejaculates into the woman's vagina will pass through the womb and into the fallopian tube until eventually one sperm reaches the egg and fertilisation will occur (see Figure 1). Once the egg is fertilised, it becomes a potential human being and begins to divide to make more and more cells. This rapidly enlarging ball of cells travels down the fallopian tube and after about one week reaches the womb and burrows into the lining of the womb. The ball of cells then forms into two separate parts: one part will develop into the baby (at this early stage it is called an embryo) and the other part develops into the afterbirth (placenta), through which food and oxygen are passed from the mother to the baby, and the membranes which form a sac containing water (liquor). The baby can then grow within the sac of waters, protected and weightless like a diver.

Over the next eight weeks the various parts of the body are formed, such as the brain, the heart, the limbs, etc., and at the end of that time in medical terms the embryo is called a foetus. This occurs about 12 weeks from the last menstrual period. A woman will now have been pregnant for ten weeks but it is easier to date back to the first day of the last menstrual period rather than to the day of ovulation, because the day of ovulation is usually not known. Pregnancy lasts on average 280 days from the first day of the last menstrual period. This is ten lunar months or nine calendar months and one week.

Pregnancy is divided into three parts known as the first, second and third trimesters. During the first trimester, up to 14 weeks, the various organs of the body are being formed. The second trimester, between 14 and 24 weeks, is the time when if the baby were born it would be too immature to survive. The third trimester is from 24 weeks until delivery, when the baby can survive if it is born alive, but its chances are generally better the longer it can stay in the womb. Thus with miscarriages we are concerned with why the pregnancy ends or the baby leaves the womb in the first and second trimesters. When a baby is born dead during or at the end of the third trimester, it is known as a stillbirth.

Miscarriage

One in five to ten conceptions ends in miscarriage. The exact number is unknown and there is evidence to suggest that, if very early miscarriages are included, the incidence may be as high as one in two. The incidence of miscarriage does not appear to have changed, and there do not appear to be significant differences between social class, although there are some racial differences; for example the type of miscarriage known as hydatidiform mole is more common in South-east Asian women. Data is far from clear, though, and offers no definite picture. Of first trimester miscarriages 50–60 per cent are genetic in origin. About 20 per cent of second trimester miscarriages are also due to genetic factors.

Genetic problems

Every cell in the human body contains 46 chromosomes, apart from the egg and the sperm, which contain 23. We have 23 chromosomes from our mother and 23 chromosomes from our father. Our chromosomes are made up of millions of genes which makes us what we are and different from everybody else. The study of genetics is the study of our genes: our inheritance from our parents. We will give half our chromosomes, and therefore half of our genes, to our children.

The egg is formed in the female ovary and the sperm in the male testicle. Part of their formation involves halving the number of chromosomes from 46 to 23 so that when the sperm fertilises the egg the correct number of chromosomes is again present. The process is complex and therefore open to error.

The 46 chromosomes are in 23 pairs; 22 of the pairs are called autosomes and one pair is the sex chromosomes responsible for maleness or femaleness. The sex choromosomes are either X or Y. Two X chromosomes make a female and one X and one Y make a male. Thus the female egg will always contain an X chromosome but the male sperm will be half X and half Y. The autosomes are responsible for other features, such as height, hair colour, etc. (see Figure 2).

During the process of fertilisation it is possible to lose a chromosome so there are only 45; this is known as monosomy. A baby developing with only one X chromosome may be born alive and apparently female and the different number of chromosomes may only be detected later when a rather short female teenager seeks medical advice because her periods never start. The problem is known medically as Turner's syndrome. The incidence of Turner's syndrome is not dependent on the age of the mother. For

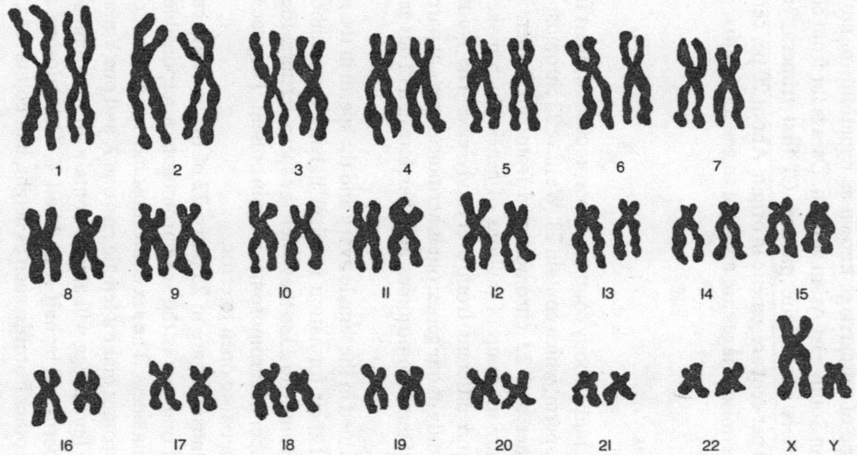

Figure 2 Normal pairs of chromosomes

every two children born with Turner's syndrome 98 per cent are miscarried. Turner's syndrome accounts for about 25 per cent of chromosomally abnormal babies, of which two thirds miscarry at about six weeks.

If a chromosome is gained, so there are 47, this is called trisomy. The best known trisomy is Down's Syndrome or Mongolism, where there are three number 21 chromosomes. Some of these trisomies are compatible with life, although the child is usually mentally defective and, apart from Down's Syndrome, does not live very long. Trisomies are also common in babies that are miscarried, accounting for 50 per cent of babies which are lost because of chromosomal abnormalities. The incidence of trisomy increases with the age of the mother and is one of the reasons why miscarriage is more common in women in their late thirties and forties.

Another problem occurs when instead of forming 46 chromosomes, 69 or 92 or other multiples of 23 are formed. This is called polyploidy and is also a cause of miscarriage for genetic reasons.

Some chromosome abnormalities do not form embryos but they may form the placenta and membranes without an embryo. In medical terms these pregnancies are referred to as 'anembryonic' pregnancies or 'blighted ovum', the ovum being another name for the fertilised egg. This can be a very difficult thing to understand and cope with; the woman feels pregnant because the placenta makes the right hormones and her emotions respond to an image of the baby developing inside, but there is no baby developing. This problem can be detected by an ultrasound scan. Ultrasound scans use very high frequency sound waves and they build up a picture from the echoes. A scan of a blighted ovum will show up the placenta and sac but no baby. Without the baby the placenta begins to die and so the pregnancy miscarries, usually six to ten weeks after the last normal period. Sometimes, however, the placenta stops growing and everything shrivels inside the womb but does not come away. The woman may be aware of feeling different, perhaps less sick, or her breasts are less tender, but still there is no bleeding, and it may not be realised that the pregnancy has failed until an ultrasound scan is performed. This situation is called a missed abortion. (The terms abortion and miscarriage are synonymous in medical usage, except in this one case where missed 'abortion' is always used.) Eventually a missed abortion will come away, but before that happens it can cause an infection of the womb or occasionally cause a disturbance of the mother's blood so it does not clot properly; therefore, once this is detected it is better to empty the womb.

One further chromosome problem leads to a strange condition called hydatidiform mole. This occurs in about one in 2,000 pregnancies in the UK. The mole is made up of an abnormal placenta consisting of thousands of small grape-like blobs. The embryo is rarely present, but can be. A woman who has a hydatidiform mole will feel very sick because the mole produces high levels of pregnancy hormones. The uterus appears to be bigger than her dates and she may have noticed bleeding from the vagina, or even seen one of the grape-like blobs pass out. Very occasionally a hydatidiform mole can become cancerous (choriocarcinoma) and so whenever it is detected the womb is emptied as soon as possible and the woman kept under medical supervision for the next year to make sure that this change does not take place. If it does, it is a treatable and usually curable form of cancer.

Genetic causes are the most common reason for a miscarriage, but unfortunately there is no treatment to prevent this from recurring. However, it does seem that avoidance of an excess of smoking cigarettes or drinking alcohol may be beneficial in providing optimal conditions for a successful pregnancy.

Because an early miscarriage tends to be due to a genetic problem, the first and second time it is usually not looked into, as it is likely to be a chance occurrence; but if it occurs a third time, the couple should have their own genetic make-up checked. Some people have an increased risk of miscarriage from genetic causes because of an abnormality in their own genetic material which does not manifest itself in themselves, but may manifest itself in the children produced by the union of genetic material from couples at risk. If such a problem is found, there is the risk of repeated miscarriages or of an abnormal baby. This problem tends to raise feelings of guilt and anger in the couple concerned. Sometimes it may be inferred that they are in some way abnormal themselves, and again the question 'why me?' will be asked. 'What have I done that may have caused this problem?' We all want a peg to hang a coat on, but with genetic problems no such peg can be found. It is again a chance happening and nothing can be done to alter the situation. Every genetic problem is individual to the couple concerned, and they should seek the advice and counselling of a genetic counsellor, who will be a specialist trained to help people understand the problem and the chance of a similar problem occurring in future pregnancies. It is advisable to see a genetic counsellor before becoming pregnant if there is a hereditary problem in the family (see p. 115)

Infections

Certain infections affecting the mother at critical times during the pregnancy can be lethal for the baby. The one which most people have heard of is rubella or German measles. This is caused by the rubella virus and if the infection occurs during the first four months of pregnancy, when the organs are being formed, then damage can occur, especially to the eyes, ears and heart. Many women have had German measles as children and therefore have their own immunity and will not get the illness again as adults. Nowadays most children are immunised against German measles. Thus the problem of German measles in pregnancy is getting less, but it still needs to be thought about. Every woman who books at an atenatal clinic in Great Britain will have a blood test to see if she is immune to German measles. If she is not she will be offered immunisation when she has delivered the baby, to protect her in subsequent pregnancies. If a woman is unfortunate enough to contract German measles in early pregnancy, there is a risk of either a spontaneous miscarriage or of the baby developing abnormally if the pregnancy continues. If this problem does arise, the couple will be carefully counselled by a doctor and termination of the pregnancy may be considered, if blood tests suggest the baby is affected. If the infection occurs after the first three months, the risk to the baby is much less.

There are other infections of the mother which can cross the placenta to affect the developing baby. The two main ones are cytomegalovirus (CMV) and toxoplasmosis. CMV is a virus which gives an influenza-like illness, usually with swollen glands. Like German measles, it is an illness most women have had as children and are thus immune to it in their adult lives. However, in similar fashion as German measles, if the infection is caught early in pregnancy, it can either cause a miscarriage or affect the developing baby. It is possible that in the future a method of immunisation for CMV will be available to schoolgirls and susceptible adult women.

Toxoplasmosis is a protozoal infection. The organism toxoplasma has a life cycle which involves more than one host. The human being usually picks up the infection by eating raw meat and from contaminated soil on unwashed fruit and vegetables or via cuts on hands when gardening. It can also be caught from infected cats if their excreta are carelessly handled. Toxoplasmosis is not common in this country but an infection in early pregnancy can cause a miscarriage or damage the developing baby. However, the likelihood of an unborn baby becoming infected is very rare (1 in 50,000 live plus stillbirths). Once an infection has occurred the woman builds up immunity for the future, so subsequent pregnancies cannot be affected. There is no immunisation against toxoplasmosis. At present screening for toxoplasmosis in the mother is unreliable and often gives information which is difficult to interpret, sometimes leading into invasive tests to the foetus which can also increase the risk of a miscarriage. Therefore current advice is of the preventative nature and includes cooking all meats well before use, taking care to wash hands and utensils when handling and storing uncooked meat, washing all meat, vegetable and salad products before eating, wearing gloves for gardening, asking someone else to change cat litter trays or wearing gloves to do so and washing hands after touching cats and kittens.

Listeriosis is an infection caused by a bacteria found widely in the environment, e.g. food products, water, soil and animal faeces. Although the disease is rare and causes only mild flu-like symptoms, it can cause miscarriage particularly in the second trimester, stillbirths or severe illness in the newborn baby. There is no single test to detect whether the infection has affected the developing baby so advice is largely preventative. Pâtes, ready-cooked chicken, soft and blue-veined cheese, goats' or ewes' milk cheeses and unpasteurised milk should be avoided during pregnancy and care should be taken to reheat ready-cooked meals thoroughly and to wash all salad and vegetable products.

Herpes is a virus infection. There are two types: one causes cold sores and the other is sexually transmitted (genital herpes) and can cause similar sores around the labia and inside the vagina, or on the man's penis. If this infection occurs for the first time in early pregnancy it may cause a miscarriage and in late pregnancy it can infect the baby born through a vagina with sores present. Thus the doctors would check the woman and if sores were present very close to the end of a pregnancy she would be advised to have a Caesarian birth.

Chickenpox, measles, mumps and influenza are all virus infections which can cause a miscarriage if the infection occurs during the first three months. It is the high temperature and severity of the generalised infection that appear to be the important factors; if the pregnancy does continue, it appears that mumps and influenza do not damage the baby. Chickenpox may be responsible for limb deformities in a baby born to a mother who has had chickenpox in the first trimester.

Other infections which cause high temperature of 38 or above may precipitate a miscarriage, especially severe kidney or chest infections. Therefore such infections need prompt medical attention and treatment with antibiotics. Other treatments such as two paracetamol tablets every four hours will help to bring down a temperature as will sponging the body with tepid water.

Syphilis is an infection which is rarely seen today but at the beginning of this century it was responsible for many miscarriages occurring in the second trimester. It seems that somehow the baby is protected in the first three months only to succumb later. Every woman in Great Britain who attends an antenatal clinic is tested for syphilis by a special blood test. This disease is readily treatable with pencillin and other antibiotics and consequently worth checking for.

Malaria may lead to foetal death and miscarriage; again, this is more likely with more severe generalised illness and high temperature.

Tuberculosis is rare in this country but, in developing countries still, the lining of the womb may become infected with TB, which will be responsible for infertility. Once the disease has been treated, however, the woman may become pregnant but has an increased risk of miscarriage.

Infections that cause abortions in farm animals

Brucellosis is a bacterial infection known to cause abortion in cattle, pigs, sheep and goats, but it is not certain whether these bacteria are responsible for miscarriage in humans. Brucellosis is being eradicated from cattle in Britain and other European countries.

Recently there has also been concern about another infection in sheep caused by the organism chlamydia psittaci and a link to spontaneous abortion in sheep farmers and veterinary surgeons working in this area. As with brucellosis, the infection is rare in humans in Great Britain and unlikely to be a problem outside the farming community. Pregnant women should avoid involvement in lambing or handling any material related to lambing. Their husbands should also take extra care with general hygiene after handling material related to lambing.

Vaginal infections

Chlamydia trachomatis is one of the most prevalent sexually transmitted bacterial infections in the world. It is often asymptomatic in women. It increases the risk of ectopic pregnancies by damaging tubal function and in pregnant women, may be associated with preterm delivery, premature rupture of membranes, low birthweight and, rarely, perinatal death. Babies born vaginally to mothers infected with chlamydia are at risk of conjunctivitis and pneumonia. Women found to have this infection, which can be diagnosed by taking a swab from the cervix, can be treated with tetracylines or azithromycin if not pregnant or with erythromycin if pregnant.

Candida (thrush) is a very common vaginal infection caused by yeasts. Trichomonas is similarly very common and caused by a protozoan. Neither appears to be linked to spontaneous miscarriage.

AIDS (Acquired Immuno Deficiency Syndrome)

The HIV virus (Human Immunosuppressive Virus) responsible for AIDS has brought a new dimension to infections and should be discussed although so far it does not appear to be linked to an increased risk of miscarriage.

By 1993, 2500 women had been found to be HIV positive. Evidence now suggests that pregnancy does not make a woman who is HIV positive more likely to progress to AIDS. The effect of HIV infection on pregnancy is more difficult to evaluate as other lifestyle factors such as smoking and drug use often confuse the results. However, there is no evidence for congenital defects, preterm labour or poor growth of the fetus in HIV-infected pregnancies. The virus can spread via the placenta to affect the baby who can be born with HIV infection. However this only happens in about 14 per cent of pregnancies in the developed world. Transmission is increased when the woman has just been infected with the virus or if she is in the later stages of HIV infection and has AIDS related complex, ARC or AIDS. Breastfeeding has been shown to increase transmission of the virus. Recent studies have shown that the antiviral drug, AZT, when given during pregnancy, may reduce the risk of transmission and that Caesarian section may also be protective.

Thus it is important that women who are at high risk of carrying the HIV virus consider having a blood test to check before becoming pregnant. If a woman is found to be HIV positive she would need to be counselled carefully and sensitively, not only about the significance of this result for her general health, but also for the implications of a pregnancy.

Drugs, cigarettes and alcohol

It is uncommon for drugs to be responsible for a miscarriage except for the very toxic drugs used in the treatment of cancer. However, there are connections between abnormalities in the developing baby and certain drugs taken during the first eight weeks of pregnancy while the baby is being formed. Alcohol is also thought to be harmful. This can be either in the form of regular social drinking or the occasional 'binge'. Cigarette smoking during pregnancy is also known to be harmful because it can effect the development of the baby's afterbirth and thus cause the developing baby to be rather small. In extreme cases this could lead to the baby dying inside the womb. It is much safer to avoid alcohol and cigarettes during pregnancy and to avoid any other drugs, especially during the first two to three months. Care should also be taken prior to conception. If you take regular tablets it is important to check with a doctor that it is safe for you to become pregnant while taking the tablets. With the majority of drugs it will be quite safe for you to continue, but occasionally you will need to change treatment befoe you try to get pregnant. In later pregnancy you may need tablets to help cope with certain symptoms common to pregnant women, but it is always worth checking with a doctor first that the medication is safe.

As for the drugs of addiction such as heroin, it appears that these may reduce fertility. They may stop ovulation or lead to a reduced sex drive. However, if an addict is carefully supervised through a pregnancy the outcome is usually successful, although the baby may have to go through several months of withdrawal after it is born, which will be supervised carefully by a paediatrician (a doctor who specialises in babies and children). Addicts are usually changed from heroin to methadone during the pregnancy and may be slowly withdrawn from drugs if they want to be, when the effects of withdrawal on the baby as well must be watched carefully.

The effect of other habit-forming drugs such as amphetamines, barbiturates and cocaine, in terms of congenital abnormalities and miscarriages, is not fully known, but it does appear that miscarriages and minor congential abnormalities such as hare lip and cleft palate and abnormalities to the limbs are more common in heavy drug abuse during early pregnancy. Crack has the same effect as cocaine. There is no proven link with miscarriages or congenital abnormalities but there is an increased risk of placental abruption, pre-term labour, premature rupture of membranes and intrauterine growth retardation. Again, other lifestyle factors such as smoking, alcohol and other drugs, may co-exist and cause problems in their own right. LSD may be associated with major abnormalities. Marijuana smoked heavily in early pregnancy may also be detrimental. The general feeling is that all these 'social drugs', including alcohol and cigarettes, are best avoided at the time of conception and during pregnancy.

X-rays

X-rays of your abdomen are best avoided in the first three months of pregnancy as in theory they may affect the developing baby. However, X-rays of other parts of your body are safe. If it is essential for you to have the X-rays, inform the doctor or dentist that you are to think you might be pregnant; they will then try to get all the information required with as few X-rays as possible. They will also protect your abdomen by giving you a lead apron to wear, which will not allow X-rays to reach that part of your body. In late pregnancy X-rays of your abdomen and pelvis are safer and may be necessary to check the size of the mother's bone structure.

Women who work in hospitals or industries with X-ray equipment or who use it at airports to check baggage should take special care to protect themselves with lead aprons and to monitor the dose of radiation they are exposed to with special badges. During the important first three months when the baby's organs are developing many women prefer not to work directly with the X-ray machinery.

Anaesthetics

As with all drugs, it is sensible to avoid an anaesthetic during the first three months of pregnancy. However, this may not always be possible. If you do need an anaesthetic, it is important to let the doctor know you might be pregnant. Most anaesthetic agents are quite safe when given for the brief period of an operation, but there does appear to be an association between miscarriage and anaesthesia, with an increased risk of miscarriages in female anaesthetists, theatre nurses and the wives of male anaesthetists. It is thought that prolonged, low-grade exposure to anaesthetic gases may be responsible. Most operating theatres nowadays are equipped with special pipes to remove waste gases and therefore minimise the risk.

Exposure to chemicals and pesticides

The evidence of research into whether exposure to toxic chemicals, pesticides and general levels of radiation in the environment and at the workplace increases the rate of miscarriage is still unclear, although it is suggested that, for instance, exposure to lead can result in impotence in men, and women who work with lead or live near a lead smelter miscarry more frequently than would be expected. When a woman who works in an industry which uses chemicals or pesticides is contemplating pregnancy it is worth her discussing this with her company's doctor or nurse and perhaps trying to transfer to another job within the firm, especially during early pregnancy. Many trade unions are now negotiating such rights for pregnant women.

Exposures to visual display units (VDUs)

There was some concern that radiation emitted from VDU screens would be harmful. Some studies indicated that women working with VDUs may be more susceptible to miscarriage than might be expected but this has not been substantiated. It is important to follow the usual recommendations for working with VDUs (e.g. not for too long at a time) during pregnancy.

Poor diet

There is no evidence linking poor diet with miscarriages. However, vitamin deficiency is associated with foetal abnormalities, in particular lack of folic acid, a B-group vitamin, is strongly linked to neural tube defects. Therefore all women have been advised to take 0.4mg of folic acid a day from the time they start trying to conceive until they are 12 weeks pregnant. Although an alteration in diet may provide this (folic acid is found in green vegetables, cereals, salads and liver) it is easier to make sure by taking it in a daily tablet. Women who have had a child with a neural tube defect or who are on anticonvulsants because they are epileptic, are advised to take a higher dose of 4mg a day for the same time period.

Health of the mother

Women who have certain other medical problems are more likely to miscarry. It appears that diabetic women, if the diabetes is not under good control at the time they conceive, are more likely to miscarry; but once the diabetes is well controlled then their chances of a miscarriage are the same as women without diabetes. This means that pre-pregnancy counselling for diabetic women and careful control of their diabetes for several months before they try to get pregnant can be very important.

If diabetes is suspected, the woman may be complaining of thirst and passing a lot of urine, and on testing, the urine will show sugar. A blood test to check sugar levels will confirm the problem. If a woman who has recently been found to be diabetic wishes to become pregnant she will need to have her blood sugar levels very well controlled to have the best chance of a successful pregnancy. The same applies to women who are already known to have diabetes. The best control of blood sugar levels is achieved with insulin injections. Therefore a diabetic woman on tablets will need to change to insulin before trying to become pregnant. Also a diabetic on insulin may well need to change her insulin injections from once a day to two or three times a day in order to achieve the perfection of sugar control necesassary to give the pregnancy the best chance.

Women who have a thyroid gland that is overproducing or underproducing thyroid hormone also need treatment to give the pregnancy the best chance of surviving. The thyroid is a gland in the neck. When it is overactive the woman loses weight, becomes anxious and has a fast pulse rate and hand tremor; she sometimes has prominent eyes. When the thyroid is underactive the woman will gain weight and become slower, her voice may become lower and her hair thinner and dry. Thyroid problems can be detected by blood tests and corrected. An overactive thyroid can usually be suppressed with tablets but sometimes the doctor may recommend surgery to remove part of the thyroid. An underactive thyroid is treated with tablets containing thyroid hormone.

Women with epilepsy should also consult their doctors before planning a pregnancy because certain tablets to control epilepsy may affect a developing baby and minor abnormalities such as a hare lip may result. Epilepsy itself is not associated with an increased risk of miscarriage.

Another medical problem is sickle cell anaemia. Women with sickle cell anaemia are usually of African or Afro-Caribbean origin. These women can have children but they do have an increased risk of miscarriage and stillbirth. Frequent blood checks for anaemia, folic acid supplements and blood transfusions throughout the pregnancy can help. It is important that all black women who become pregnant are tested for sickle cell anaemia.

Women who have other medical problems such as high blood pressure, kidney or heart disease will also need careful counselling before becoming pregnant. Not only may there be a risk of late miscarriage but also the pregnancy may be detrimental to the health of the woman. A particular problem can occur with autoimmune diseases where the body produces antibodies to its own tissues as part of the disease process. The presence of anti-phospholipid antibodies comprise a family of auto-antibodies which have a well-established association with foetal loss both within the first and second trimester and later on in pregnancy as stillbirths. The exact way in which the presence of these antibodies causes foetal loss is not known although it is thought to cause blockage in the placental blood flow. The best treatment is not known either and may range from no treatment to a combination of Heparin, Aspirin, or Steroids. Clinical trials are still underway.

Obviously there are many medical problems that can affect a woman in the childbearing years and each illness will affect individuals differently. It is impossible to generalise on such a large subject. However, it is always best to seek counselling before the pregnancy. It is very unusual for doctors to counsel against a pregnancy, but it may mean altering treatments or coming into hospital for rest in early pregnancy. Some hospitals now have special clinics called Pre-pregnancy Advisory Clinics, where advice on such problems will be offered. Otherwise a woman should discuss the problem with the doctor looking after her medical problem, her GP or local obstetrician.

Pregnancy with a coil in the womb

A pregnancy occurring with a coil (IUCD) inside the womb is by defintion a contraceptive failure. Many such pregnancies continue without problems but some have bleeding through the pregnancy and there is an increased tendency to miscarriage, premature rupture of the membranes and premature labour and an increased risk of infection. If a woman becomes pregnant with a coil in the womb, the doctor will try to remove the coil early in pregnancy if the strings are still visible. If the strings are not visible the coil is best left alone.

This is a problem that can cause a woman considerable anxiety. She may feel that she cannot cope with the pregnancy continuing and thus seek a termination of pregnancy, with all the feelings of guilt that this may raise, however much she feels she could not cope with a baby who may have been affected. She may have had these ambivalent feelings but opt to continue the pregnancy only to miscarry the baby after.

There is also a risk that a pregnancy occurring with a coil in place may be an ectopic pregnancy. If a woman ever finds herself pregnant with a coil in place, it is wise to seek medical advice early and to be examined internally. The doctor can help to make the choice that is right for each woman, although the final decision is hers alone. If she wishes to continue the pregnancy, an ultrasound scan can be arranged if there is any doubt about an ectopic pregnancy. If the coil threads are visible, it is advisable to have the coil removed. There is a small risk that this will precipitate a miscarriage but the risk is greater if the coil is left.

Multiple pregnancy

Multiple pregnancy rates vary worldwide. In the UK the rate for twins is about 1 in 80 pregnancies although this may have increased recently with the use of assisted reproductive techniques, such as

IVF. Miscarriage occurs more frequently in multiple pregnancy than in singleton pregnancy as does pre-term (i.e. before 37 weeks) labour, which may occur up to eight times more frequently in multiple pregnancies. The length of pregnancy decreases as the number of foetuses present increases.

Sometimes if the uterus is overstretched, it will go into labour too early. This can occur in a multiple pregnancy and it is then a matter of timing the labour to prevent the babies being born too early when they are unable to survive; if they are born a little later, with intensive care in an incubator they may survive.

It may be possible to prevent a miscarriage with twins by admitting the mother to hospital and stopping the contractions of the uterus with a salbutamol or ritrodrine drip. Once the contractions have subsided the mother can come off the drip and take salbutamol or ritrodrine tablets. However, it is not always possible to stop the contractions, especially if the cervix is opening, and in such an event miscarriages will be inevitable. This can be distressing, as often the babies are fairly big and perfectly formed.

If a previous twin pregnancy has miscarried, then in the next pregnancy an early ultrasound scan will help to show whether the mother has twins again. It may also be helpful to come into hospital for rest about the time of previous miscarriage and also to take salbutamol or ritrodrine tablets, which help to relax the muscle of the uterus.

Recurrent miscarriage

The cause for recurrent (three or more) miscarriages is often not found. Possible causes can be genetic, hormonal or immunological, maternal illness or infection, abnormalities of the uterus or cervix or rhesus incompatability. It could be that different miscarriages are due to different precipitating factors.

Usually the couple will need to be investigated selectively, depending on the likely cause of the miscarriages as determined by taking details of the miscarriages themselves, medical details of the couple and their family medical histories and also examining both partners. Investigations could include chromosome analysis, HLA antigen testing, blood grouping and checking for rhesus antibodies, hormone estimates and hysterosalpingogram (see p. 84) to check for abnormalities of the shape of the uterus or cervical canal.

The different treatments available are outlined in the relevant sections. It must be remembered that where no cause is found, the chance of a successful pregnancy is still between 50 and 70 per cent, depending on the individual woman's own situation, and that even where treatments are available the odds may not be greatly improved and 100 per cent success can never be achieved.

Abnormal shape of the womb and fibroids

The shape of the uterus may be altered by fibroids, which are balls of muscle tissue within the muscular wall of the uterus; if the fibroid distorts the cavity of the uterus, this may affect the ability of the uterus to carry the pregnancy successfully. Fibroids are more common in women over 30 and women of African and African-Caribbean origin.

The uterus itself may have developed abnormally. In the female embryo the uterus is formed by two separate tubes fusing together, but this fusion may have not have been complete. These different shapes of the uterus are associated with miscarriages that occur in the second trimester. The commonest abnormality is a bircornuate (two horned) uterus (see Figure 3).

The problem will be suspected if there are recurrent miscarriages. The shape of the cavity of the uterus can then be checked by a special X-ray called an HSG. This X-ray involves having an internal examination. The doctor uses a metal speculum to open the vagina and see the cervix. (This is the same instrument that is used to see the cervix when a cervical smear is taken.) A special liquid is then injected into the uterus. This liquid shows up on X-rays and will therefore outline the shape of the cavity.

This X-ray can be painful and cause cramping, similar to period pains, as the liquid is injected. If this happens, the doctor can give some pain-killing tablets and a short rest is advised before going home. It is sensible to come with a friend to escort you home.

If a fibroid or septum is found to be distorting the cavity of the uterus, the doctor may recommend an operation to correct the abnormality. This can be done by a telescopic instrument inserted through the cervix called a hysteroscope. Large fibroids may be removed before pregnancy by an abdominal operation called myomectomy. Usually fibroids do not distort the cavity of the womb and are therefore best left alone unless they are very big.

If the uterus is bicornuate, the doctor will usually advise against an operation. Very occasionally, however, an operation is done to

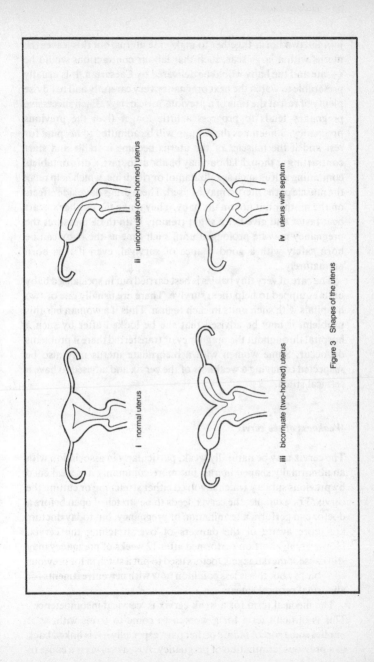

i normal uterus

ii unicornuate (one-horned) uterus

iii bicornuate (two-horned) uterus

iv uterus with septum

Figure 3   Shapes of the uterus

join the two horns together to make one uterus, but this leaves the uterus with a large scar, such that labour contractions would be unsafe and the baby would be delivered by Caesarian. It is usually preferable to watch the next pregnancy very carefully and to advise plenty of rest at the time of a previous miscarriage. Each successive pregnancy tends to progress a little longer than the previous pregnancy. Sometimes the woman will be admitted to hospital for rest and if the muscles of the uterus become irritable and start contracting as though labour may be about to start, a drip or tablets containing a drug such as salbutamol or ritodrine, which help relax the muscle of the uterus, may be used. These drugs have side effects on the mother but not on the baby. They make the mother's heart beat faster and give her a slight tremor. With these measures the pregnancy may be prolonged until such time as the baby can be born safely with a good chance of survival, even if it is born prematurely.

The care of very tiny babies is best carried out in specialised baby units equipped to help them survive. There are usually one or two hospitals with such units in each region. Thus if a woman has this problem, it may be advised that she be looked after by such a hospital throughout the pregnancy or transferred there if problems do occur. Some women with a bicornuate uterus may also be suspected of having a weakness of the cervix and advised to have a cervical stitch.

Weakness of the cervix

The cervix may be naturally weak, particularly in association with an abnormally shaped uterus, but more commonly it is weakened by previous surgery which involved either stretching or cutting the cervix. For example, the cervix needs to be stretched open before a doctor can perform a termination of pregnancy, but today doctors are more aware of the dangers of overstretching the cervix. However, an abortion performed after 12 weeks of pregnancy may still cause some damage. Doctors used to put a stitch in for previous cone biopsy but this is less common now with newer treatments for abnormal cervical smears.

The medical term for a weak cervix is 'cervical incompetence'. This is difficult term for a woman to come to terms with, as it implies some sort of failure on her part, especially if it is linked back to a previous termination of pregnancy. A weak cervix is a cause of miscarriage after the fourth month of pregnancy when the increasing weight of the pregnancy on the cervix may cause it to open too early. As the cervix opens the membranes bulge through. Usually the mother is aware of the waters breaking first. This is followed by a short labour.

The treatment in a subsequent pregnancy is to put a special stitch into the cervix (see Figure 4). This is called either a Shriodkar or Macdonald suture. This is done in hospital under a general or epidural anaesthetic at about 14–16 weeks of pregnancy (which is after the time that most genetic problems would have already miscarried). The stitch is put around the cervix like a purse string. The woman may be kept resting in hospital for a day or two after the operation. The stitch is usually removed during the thirty-eighth week of pregnancy, not under general anaesthetic, as it is much easier to take out than to put in.

Usually the woman is advised against sexual intercourse with penetration if she has a stitch in, and she will be counselled that all other forms of lovemaking are all right. Most women who have had a late miscarriage will avoid intercourse about the time they miscarried previously, although there seems to be no evidence for or against it being a cause; however, the above advice helps take away the guilt of linking sex with a further miscarriage should this occur. About the time of a previous miscarriage the woman would also be advised to avoid reaching orgasm, as the uterus contracts after orgasm and the contractions could affect the stitch.

Inserting a cervical stitch cannot guarantee 100 per cent that premature labour will not occur; there is no rule that can show how different women will react to it. Sometimes the stich can cause infection and inflammation that may lead to premature labour, but then that might have occurred anyway. Sometimes the stitch can lead to scar tissue forming around the cervix which may slow dilatation of the cervix, resulting in a longer labour, and possibly necessitate a Caesarian delivery. However, in assessing the possible risks of inserting a stitch, one needs to remember that the outcome should be a healthy baby delivered at full term.

The rhesus problem

Everyone has a certain blood group, which is A, B, O or AB. There is another blood group which is known as rhesus; 85 per cent of the population are rhesus positive and 15 per cent are rhesus negative.

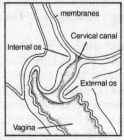

membranes

Cervical canal

Internal os

External os

Vagina

The 'normal' cervix at
about 16 weeks of pregnancy

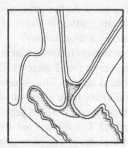

An 'incompetent' cervix
in the early stages. The
internal os has opened

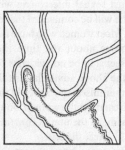

If a stitch is not inserted,
the external os will open
and the membranes bulge
through the cervix

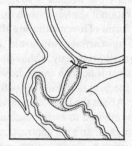

A cervical stitch in place

Figure 4   Cervical 'incompetence' and the cervical stitch

If a person who is blood group A receives a blood transfusion from someone who is blood group B, for the first transfusion they will be all right, but their body will form antibodies to blood group B and these antibodies will react with the next transfusion and destroy all the transfused blood group B. This is why it is important to cross-match blood before giving a blood tranfusion. It is also important to cross-match for rhesus antibodies.

With pregnancy the rhesus problem occurs when the mother is rhesus negative and the baby is rhesus positive. The first time a rhesus negative mother carries a rhesus positive baby there should be no problem, but at the moment of the baby's birth some of its rhesus positive blood may pass into the mother's blood. The mother will form antibodies to rhesus positive blood such that in a subsequent pregnancy with a rhesus positive baby the antibodies to rhesus positive blood will cross the placenta from the mother to the baby and destroy the baby's blood cells, making it anaemic. Usually the first time this occurs the baby is only mildly affected and may require a blood transfusion after it is born, but in subsequent pregnancies the baby may be severely affected and may need to be transfused while still inside the womb. However, very severely affected babies die within the first five to six months and are miscarried, or the pregnancy is terminated once the baby's death has been confirmed.

Since the early 1970s it has been possible to reduce the rhesus problem considerably by giving an injection to a rhesus negative woman after a miscarriage, ectopic pregnancy, termination of pregnancy or childbirth itself. The injection is called Anti-D. The gene responsible for the rhesus positive factor is called Big D. Absence of Big D is rhesus negative or Little d. Everyone has two rhesus genes, one from each parent. A rhesus negative person is dd, a rhesus positive person can be DD or Dd. At the time of childbirth or miscarriage, etc., it is possible for rhesus positive blood cells from the baby to cross into the mother's circulation. (If the baby is rhesus negative there is no problem.) As mentioned earlier, the mother will form antibodies to D called Anti-D and these will destroy the rhesus positive blood cells. However, it takes about three days before the mother forms her own antibodies; thus if she is given an injection of Anti-D before this happens, the Anti-D injected will destroy the rhesus positive cells and the mother will not form antibodies.

The problem, however, has not completely disappeared. Sometimes a woman who miscarried before Anti-D injections became available may have problems with subsequent pregnancies and sometimes the mother is sensitised by the baby's blood cells crossing into her blood stream before labour rather than during labour. All rhesus negative women have three to four blood checks during pregnancy to look for antibodies. Once antibodies have formed, subsequent pregnancies may be complicated, as explained earlier. The severity of the problem does depend on the partner's blood group. If the father is DD, all the babies will have rhesus positive Dd because every sperm will carry the D gene; but if he is Dd, half the babies will be rhesus positive and half will be rhesus negative. It is therefore important to know if the father is DD or Dd. If the problem is severe and the father is DD, it is better for the couple not to attempt a further pregnancy. Some couples can come to terms with AID (artificial insemination by donor) when the semen comes from a rhesus negative donor. If the partner is Dd, there is 50:50 chance of the baby being rhesus negative and the pregnancy progressing normally. However, if the baby is rhesus positive, it is likely that the pregnancy will again end in miscarriage.

Immunological problems

In the same way that everyone has a certain blood group we also have different tissue types, and these are responsible for our ability to accept organ transplants from another individual. Thus if a person requires a kidney transplant, their tissue is typed and they have to wait for a suitable kidney from a donor with a similar tissue type. This will reduce the risk of the kidney being rejected. Tissue types depend on human lymphocytic antigens (HLA). Lymphocytes are special white blood cells that fight certain types of infections and are involved in tissue rejection with organ transplantation. These antigens are genetically determined and found in most tissues.

In many ways the developing foetus is like a transplant organ with many different HLA antigens and yet the mother's uterus does not reject this different tissue, a fact which has interested doctors for a long time. It now appears that it is beneficial for the foetus to have many different HLA antigens from the mother, as this seems to stimulate a special response in the mother that allows the foetus to develop. If the mother and father have similar HLA antigens the mother and foetus will have similar antigens and this seems to prevent the stimulation of necessary protective substances.

Research has shown that couples with a history of recurrent miscarriages are more likely to have similar HLA tissue types. Various approaches have been tried to overcome this. The woman can have infusions of special donor white blood cells, or injections of her partner's white blood cells, into the skin of her forearm before and during early pregnancy. Both techniques have had some success in achieving a successful pregnancy. However, two factors must be borne in mind when considering the results of these new techniques.

First, pregnancies following recurrent miscarriages in the first trimester have about a 70 per cent chance of a successful outcome with no treatment at all, and these techniques only improve the outcome a little, to about 78 per cent. Second, of the recorded ongoing pregnancies following this treatment, there has been a higher incidence of premature and small-for-dates babies with an increased risk of stillbirth or neonatal death. Thus the treatment is not without possible problems and couples need to be carefully and realistically counselled beforehand.

Hormone imbalance

The part played by hormones in maintaining a pregnancy has long been in dispute. The two female hormones oestrogen and progesterone have both been given to women who have repeated early miscarriages to try to save the pregnancy. The hormone oestrogen was very popular in the USA in the 1950s but in the 1970s it was realised that there was a link between this treatment with synthetic oestrogens and vaginal cancer in young women who had been exposed to this hormone when they were inside their mother's womb.

The hormone progesterone has been used far more widely because it has long been considered the most important hormone in maintaining a pregnancy, and low progesterone levels in early pregnancy are associated with miscarriages caused by chromosomal abnormalities. Critical studies examining the effect of progesterone and comparing the effect of a placebo ('sugar pill') showed no difference in the outcome, and it appears that the main benefit is in the reassurance and psychological support that 'something is being done'. It has been argued that progestogen preparations (synthetic tablets similar to progesterone) will do no harm so why not give them 'just in case', but this is not altogether true, because some progestogens have been shown to affect the developing labia and clitoris of a baby girl, making them appear more like a baby boy's scrotum and penis.

High baseline levels of the pituitary hormone LH, such as found in polycystic ovarian disease (PCO) have been associated with early pregnancy loss. Current trials are looking into ways of reducing the LH levels in early pregnancy. Women who have polycystic ovarian syndrome are at increased risk of early miscarriage and it seems that losing weight helps reduce this risk. This is probably because it helps redress the hormone imbalance which is present in this condition.

Ectopic Pregnancy

An ectopic pregnancy is a pregnancy that starts to grow outside the womb. Usually this occurs in the fallopian tube (see Figure 5). The incidence of ectopic pregnancy is about one in 300 conceptions. There is some evidence to suggest that this is increasing. A fair proportion of ectopic pregnancies occur for no reason in healthy fallopian tubes, but the rest occur in already damaged fallopian tubes, which slow down the progress of the fertilised egg from the tube to the uterus. The fertilised egg is more likely, therefore, to try to grow in the tube before the friendly environment of the womb is reached.

Various factors may damage the fallopian tube. Usually the damage is from infections which may come from outside the tube, such as from a burst appendix, or from an infection in the womb which spreads up inside the tube. This can occur when there is infection after an incomplete miscarriage or after termination of pregnancy. There is an increased evidence of infection in women using the coil for contraceptive purposes. Another group of infections are sexually transmitted: gonorrhoea and chlamydia (the chief organism responsible for non specific urethritis – NSU) are the most common problems. An infection in the fallopian tube is known as salpingitis.

An ectopic pregnancy is more likely to occur in a fallopian tube which was previously blocked and then reopened by tubal surgery and has also been known to occur in a tube after sterilisation. The risk of pregnancy following female sterilisation is around one in 500–1,000; of these about 20 per cent will be ectopic. There may also be a slightly increased risk of ectopic pregnancy in women

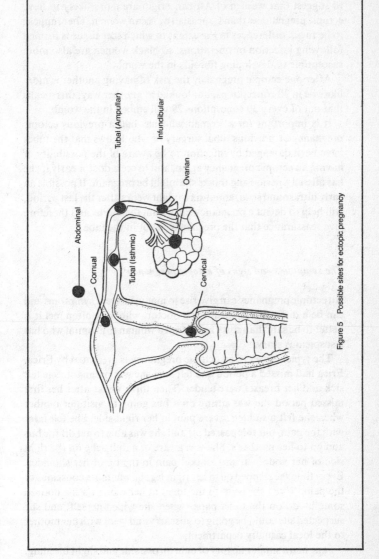

Figure 5   Possible sites for ectopic pregnancy

taking the progesterone-only contraceptive pill. There is some data to suggest that women of African origin are more likely to have ectopic pregnancies than Caucasian or Asian women. There appear to be racial differences in the extent to which scar tissue is formed following infection or operations, so black women are also more susceptible to developing fibroids in the womb.

After one ectopic pregnancy the risk of having another is more like one in 30 conceptions, but looked at another way, this means that out of every 30 conceptions 29 will embed in the womb.

It is important for a woman who has had a previous ectopic pregnancy or previous tubal surgery or who knows that the tubes have been damaged by infection to be aware of the possibility of having an ectopic pregnancy again, and to see a doctor early if she has missed a period and thinks she might be pregnant. If possible an early ultrasound scan, about six to eight weeks after the last period, will help to detect a pregnancy sac within the uterus and therefore give reassurance that the pregnancy is not in the tube.

The symptoms and signs of ectopic pregnancy

An ectopic pregnancy can give rise to many different symptoms and can be a difficult diagnosis for a doctor, who may often feel it is better to be safe than sorry and admit a woman to hospital who has a suspicious story.

The typical story of an ectopic pregnancy is presented by Erica. Erica had missed a period and felt sure she was pregnant. She felt sick and her breasts were tender. Then three weeks after her first missed period she was sitting on a bus going to visit her mother when she felt a sudden severe pain in her right side. She felt faint with the pain, but this passed off and she was able to get off the bus and go to her mother's. She was aware of a dull ache on the right side of her abdomen and an odd pain in the tip of her shoulder. Every time she stepped on to her right leg she was more conscious of the pain. When she went to the toilet at her mother's she noticed some blood on the toilet paper when she wiped herself, and she suspected she could be going to miscarry and went with her mother to the local casualty department.

Jane had a similar history of pain on one side and slight bleeding. Over the next two weeks she experienced two further episodes of pain and feeling faint and finally she had an episode of severe pain and collapsed at home. Her husband called an emergency ambulance and she was taken immediately to hospital.

What had in fact been happening was that the pregnancy had begun to grow in the tube and the tube had been stretched. If the pregnancy grows in the narrow part of the tube close to the womb then problems will start earlier because the tube cannot stretch as much as the wider part close to the ovary. Once the tube becomes stretched it may split and blood will leak into the woman's abdomen causing sudden pain and a feeling of faintness. Some of this blood may track upwards if she lies down and this will irritate the diaphragm, which is the big muscle dividing the abdomen from the chest. The nerve supplying the diaphragm also supplies the shoulder and thus pain coming from the diaphragm is interpreted as pain in the tip of the shoulder.

Once blood begins to leak the pregnancy itself dies and the hormone levels in the woman's body fall. The woman may notice she feels less sick and her breasts are less tender. This drop in the hormone level also affects the lining of the womb, which has been responding as if the pregnancy were developing in the right place. The lining of the womb therefore begins to break down and bleeding from the vagina occurs.

Sometimes after one or two warning leaks the tube completely bursts. However, this emergency may occur without any warning. When this happens the woman bleeds heavily internally. She will collapse with sudden severe pain on one side which spreads across the abdomen, she feels faint and looks pale and sweaty. This situation is an emergency and can indeed be life threatening. The woman needs urgent hospital attention and surgery to stop the internal bleeding. It is because of the danger of such an emergency that doctors treat any suspicion of an ectopic pregnancy seriously and would advise that the woman comes into hospital. An ultrasound scan may help give the answer, but not always. When there is still doubt an operation to look into the abdomen, called a laparoscopy (see pp. 104–6), will be advised.

If the pregnancy is developing in the narrow part of the tube symptoms will become evident early, usually just after a missed period, up to six weeks from the last period or three to four weeks from fertilisation. The wider the part of the tube that the ectopic pregnancy is growing in, the later it can start to show symptoms. Thus, if it is developing in the wide part of the tube, the ampulla, it may not be suspected that the pregnancy is ectopic until ten weeks from a missed period. It is also possible for the ectopic pregnancy to show up even later, after three to four or even more months. When this occurs it usually means that the embryo/foetus has died and the pregnancy tissue has ceased to grow but has become organised into a mass within the tube. This is somewhat similar to the missed abortion situation in the uterus.

The very dramatic ruptured ectopics tend to be those that show up early where the pregnancy is growing in the narrow part of the tube. This is because if the tube ruptures it is closer to major blood vessels, especially the main uterine artery. An ectopic pregnancy in the ampulla can spontaneously 'abort' into the peritoneal cavity and be absorbed in time.

There are various other problems that can mimic an ectopic pregnancy. For example, a pregnancy in the womb that is miscarrying can sometimes cause pain more on one side than the other. An infection around the fallopian tubes (salpingitis) can cause pain and upset the regular period cycle. An ovarian cyst can also upset the period cycle and can cause pain on one side if the cyst twists or bursts.

The Hospital Experience

Fran Reader

Revised by Fran Reader
and Kirsten Duckitt

The hospital experience will be a very individual affair depending on many factors, such as how advanced the pregnancy is, and how busy the casualty, ward and theatre staff are. But whatever the physical experience, for most women who miscarry it is a profound emotional experience.

Hospitals, doctors and nurses vary, but they are almost always busy places and busy people. However, somewhere out of the bureaucracy, the pressure of work, and the lack of funds, there should still be time to treat each woman experiencing a miscarriage as an individual, with care and sensitivity; to answer her questions honestly and to advise on the future. Why is it, therefore, that frequently the hospital experience is so cold and confusing? Once in hospital, you appear to become a number, away from your own patch, vulnerable in your nightdress and not suffering from anything that the doctors and nurses can 'cure'.

The business of miscarriage is depressing for medical staff; they rarely have anything positive to offer, they feel 'impotent'. The answers to questions may appear cold and unfeeling: 'I don't know why you are miscarrying'; I cannot give you anything to stop you miscarrying'; I advise you to rest, but that will not necessarily stop you miscarrying'; 'This is a very common problem – it happens to about one in five women who become pregnant'; 'I cannot promise you it will never happen again'.

In a typical busy district hospital two to three women experiencing miscarriage will be seen every day of the year. For each woman it is an extremely personal event – it has probably never happened to her before. For the doctors and nurses on a gynaecology ward, it is one of the commonest problems they are involved with. Frequently the woman is admitted to hospital at night when the young junior doctor may be short on sleep and short on the ability to offer emotional support. Apart from the pressure of work, many other emotional factors can be involved in the personal lives of the doctors and nurses involved in the care of a woman miscarrying. For everyone, man and woman, the area of pregnancy is bound up in emotions and we all have different expectations, both doctors of patients and patients of doctors, depending on our own social background and previous life experiences.

During my involvement with this book, I initially felt that I was not listening properly or counselling with sufficient thought and sensitivity. I therefore resolved to 'do better'. However, I found that a blanket approach of in-depth counselling to every woman who miscarried was not always welcome and at the same time I exhausted myself emotionally and physically as the couselling added time to my already busy schedule. I also found my involvement with miscarriage led to feelings of resentment about women requesting abortion counselling and dampened the joy I used to share with women giving birth successfully. Thus, like a pendulum, I swung back to a more middle-of-the-road approach so that I could work with each woman individually, keeping myself more detached from her grief but at the same time still caring. I now try to differentiate between women who need in-depth counselling and those who don't. I find I have developed certain phrases I use for most women and I hope they still sound sincere, because they are. I then elaborate or not, depending on which approach I sense to be appropriate.

Feelings about the role as a woman doctor can also affect our ability to listen and counsel effectively. For example, before I had children I knew that there was a clash between my desire to further my career and my desire to be pregnant. At this time I found it hard not to let jealousy colour my approach to pregnant women. Later on, during pregnancy, the physical fact of being pregnant also led to being embarrassed at times when working with women who were experiencing a loss of their own pregnancy. Similar feelings have been expressed by other female colleagues, such as a ward sister who had experienced problems of infertility. Emotional reactions are not confined to women – a young male colleague described a time when he recognised in himself a problem with coping with women's tears at work as he was in the process of separating from his wife and couldn't cope with her tears on his nights off duty. He was feeling a failure at work and at home and needed to accept his own tears.

When I first wrote along these lines, I sensed some criticism for asking for understanding for the doctors and nurses when the book was about improving the understanding of couples' and especially women's experiences of miscarriage. However, I feel it is important to fit the problem into the context of today's society, medical and nursing training and all personal interactions. I have considered some of the possible answers to the dilemmas in the section on the future at the end of this chapter. The next sections will, I hope, help to explain and demystify some of the hospital procedures that may be encountered.

Arrival at the Hospital

The woman may be seen in casualty or the GP may refer her directly to the gynaecology ward. On arrival in hospital, a nurse will check the woman's pulse, blood pressure and temperature, and assess the degree of urgency on the basis of the woman's overall condition, pain and bleeding, etc. Most casualty departments are busy and a period of waiting is not unusual. Very ill people are seen first, and rightly so, but this can also add to the waiting time.

The first doctor to see a woman who is miscarrying is usually the duty doctor, on call for gynaecology. He or she may be in training for a career in general practice or a hospital speciality. The next doctor called is usually a junior doctor specialising in gynaecology. Sometimes he or she will be the first doctor called and, depending on this doctor's experience in dealing with miscarriages, he or she may call a senior doctor.

The doctor usually takes a detailed history of the woman's general health and past and present pregnancies and examines her to check her general health and ensure she is fit for a general anaesthetic should this be required. An internal examination is important to see if the womb is the right size for the dates of pregnancy, to check if the neck of the womb (cervix) is closed or open, or, if an ectopic pregnancy is suspected, to see if there is a tender swelling to either the right or the left of the uterus. A vaginal examination will not cause a miscarriage, although if the woman does miscarry soon after, it is easy to understand how the cause and effect could be linked in her mind. Therefore, if a woman is really afraid of being examined and if there is only minimal bleeding, the doctor may defer the examination and arrange an ultrasound scan of the womb instead.

As part of the examination the doctor may wish to look at the cervix using a metal speculum to help hold open the vagina. There may be discharge suggesting infection and if this is the case the doctor will take swabs from the cervix to check for this. After the examination a blood test is taken to check for anaemia, the blood-clotting mechanism if this is relevant, and the woman's blood group in case she needs a blood transfusion and also because women who are rhesus negative need an injection of Anti-D after a miscarriage or ectopic pregnancy. Other investigations that may be organised include a pregnancy test on a urine specimen and an ultrasound scan to check whether the pregnancy is or is not continuing. Sometimes a woman with a threatened miscarriage or possible ectopic pregnancy comes to the antenatal clinic and will be examined there instead by the doctor and admitted to the ward if necessary.

If the woman's partner is with her, the doctor will ask the woman if she wants her partner to be present during the examination. All male doctors will be chaperoned by a nurse, unless the partner remains present during the examination.

If a woman is admitted to a ward from the casualty or antenatal department, her experience will obviously vary depending on the stage of the miscarriage or ectopic pregnancy and also on the length of the pregnancy so far. Most women experiencing an early miscarriage or ectopic pregnancy will be cared for on a gynaecology ward, whereas a later miscarriage may be cared for in the obstetric department.

Some hospitals now have a walk-in early pregnancy problem clinic where pregnancy tests, scans etc can be organised.

Treatment for a Threatened Miscarriage

If a miscarriage is threatened, it is common to suggest rest as the only treatment, but even rest is not the answer, although it often helps psychologically to think 'I did everything possible'. A threatened miscarriage will usually be diagnosed after an ultra-sound scan, which shows that the pregnancy is continuing despite the bleeding. This situation can cause a lot of anxiety, not only because it is still possible to miscarry but also because of the concern that if the pregnancy does continue then the baby may be abnormal. However, this is not usually the case – if the bleeding does settle, then the majority of pregnancies continue successfully. If an embryo with a heart beat is seen on the scan, then the majority (94 per cent) of such pregnancies will continue. It is not uncommon in this situation to see a second sac which is empty. This suggests that the bleeding is coming from the early loss of one baby of a twin pregnancy. The sac containing the live embryo continues to develop normally.

Sometimes in early pregnancy, when there is bleeding, the ultrasound scan can be ambivalent, especially if only a sac can be seen in the uterus and not the foetus. After six and a half weeks the scan should be able to pick up the foetal echoes and heart beat, maybe even at five and a half weeks if the scan is performed transvaginally. If the scan shows a sac the size of a six-week pregnancy, when the foetus should be further advanced, this could mean a missed abortion or else a successful pregnancy but not as far on as the dates suggest. This can usually be resolved by having another scan one to two week later. If the sac has not grown then a missed abortion is confirmed. The week of waiting can be very frustrating and frightening, especially if at the end of the week the news is not good. It is usually not necessary to stay in hospital during this week.

A threatened miscarriage in later pregnancy, for example at 20 weeks, usually means the woman resting in an antenatal ward, which can be distressing if other women are successfully having their babies, but there may be other women with similar problems and generally women do help one another and spontaneously provide a support group in this situation.

Treatment for an Inevitable or Incomplete Miscarriage

If a miscarriage is inevitable or incomplete, there is likely to be more pain and bleeding than with a threatened miscarriage. The pain can be severe and the bleeding heavy and frightening, particularly in second-trimester miscarriages. There is also the fear of passing the baby and of being helpless to do anything.

When a miscarriage is inevitable or incomplete in the first trimester it is usual for arrangements to be made for an operation to be performed to empty the womb under general anaesthetic. This operation is called an ERPC. The doctor may describe this operation as a D and C. Another term for this operation is 'having a scrape of the womb'. These terms actually apply to the non-pregnant uterus but as most women know about a D and C and a 'scrape', a doctor may keep to these terms when describing the operation.

If there is heavy bleeding, it may be necessary to give an anaesthetic and perform the operation as an emergency, but usually there is a delay while waiting for the operating theatre to be free, or because the woman has recently had something to eat or drink, in which case it is preferable to wait at least four and usually six hours before giving an anaesthetic. This ensures that the stomach is empty and thus reduces the risk of vomiting while under the anaesthetic. Vomiting can be dangerous if acid stomach contents get into the lungs. In an emergency situation anaesthetists have methods of coping with this potential problem.

A pain-killing injection such as pethidine is given if necessary; this helps to dull cramping pains. If there is heavy bleeding another injection may be necessary to help the womb contract. This injection is ergometrine or syntocinon, which sometimes have the side effect of causing vomiting, but their effect on controlling bleeding is very important. They work by causing strong contractions in the womb. A third injection to help control vomiting may be given. All these injections do have a purpose and can be very helpful in what is already a distressing situation. If the bleeding is heavy it is important for the woman to have an intravenous drip. Sometimes it may be necessary to give a blood transfusion. In order to control heavy bleeding, it may also be necessary for a doctor to examine the woman vaginally to see if any of the pregnancy tissue is sitting in the cervix, holding it open and thus increasing pain and further bleeding. When this is found, the doctor can remove the tissue with her fingers or, by using a speculum to see the cervix, gently remove the tissue with forceps. This may all sound painful and difficult for a woman to cope with, but it can be an extremely important procedure and once the tissue is free from the cervix the pain and bleeding ease off.

Before an ERPC several procedures are necessary for safety. Nail varnish and make-up are removed so that the anaesthetist can observe the colour of the nails and lips while the woman is under the anaesthetic. Jewellery that can be taken off is removed so that accidental injury does not occur, and jewellery that cannot be removed is secured with tape.

The anaesthetist usually sees the woman before the operation and will ask questions to make sure there are no allergies to drugs that may be used. Any information about a previous anaesthetic is helpful. It is also important to remove any false teeth and for the anaesthetist to know about crowns or loose teeth, etc. The operation is explained by a doctor and a consent form for the anaesthetic and operation is signed. For an ERPC the anaesthetist puts the woman to sleep with an injection into a vein in the back of the hand. The woman is then kept asleep during the operation by a combination of further intravenous drugs and by breathing gases, which the anaesthetist gives her via a mask held over the nose and mouth. Because the woman will be asleep after the injection she is unaware of the mask over her face.

When she is asleep the woman's legs are placed in special stirrups – this is called the lithotomy position. The doctor wears a special sterile gown and gloves and cleans the woman's bottom and vagina and drapes the area with sterile towels so that the whole procedure is clean and sterile, reducing the risk of infection. With an inevitable or incomplete miscarriage the neck of the womb is open and the doctor can gently scrape the lining of the womb clean. The womb often feels very soft and the doctor operates very carefully and gently as it is possible to perforate the uterus in this soft state. (If this rare complication does occur the doctor may wish to open up the abdomen and stitch the womb to prevent any haemorrhage. Very rarely, it is necessary to perform a hysterectomy – removal of the uterus.) With a missed abortion, as the cervix is closed, it is gently dilated open before the womb is scraped clean – sometimes a special suction apparatus is used to empty the womb rather than scraping it. Because the womb is soft and the doctor is very gentle and careful during an ERPC, occasionally all the pregnancy tissue inside the womb is not removed at the first operation. Unfortunately this may mean a further ERPC is necessary if the woman continues to have further pain and bleeding. This is an unfortunate complication but it is not as serious as perforation of the uterus, which is after all what the doctor is trying to avoid.

With a later inevitable miscarriage the experience is even more like labour and the woman may well be looked after in a labour ward or gynaecology ward. She will be offered pain relief in one of three ways. She can have strong pain-killing injections, or the same pain-killing drugs delivered by a continuous transfusion. She can control the rate of this transfusion within preset safety limits. This is known as patient-controlled analgesia (PCA). Finally, she can have an epidural. An anacsthetist will put in the epidural. A fine plastic catheter is introduced into space called the epidural space in the lower back. Nerves which carry the sensation of pain from the uterus to the spinal cord run through this space. The anaesthetist first puts local anaesthetic into the skin of the lower back to numb the skin and then pushes a needle, through which the plastic catheter can be threaded, into the epidural space and then the needle is removed. More local anaesthetic can be injected, from time to time during the labour, through the catheter to bathe the nerves. This takes away the pain coming from the womb.

Quite often with a later miscarriage the baby and the placenta come away completely, leaving the uterus empty; an injection called syntometrine, given after the baby is delivered, helps to expel the placenta. Sometimes the placenta does not come away and an anaesthetic is then required so that the doctor can empty the womb. This can be done under the epidural if this has been working satisfactorily during the labour. The epidural is topped up to give sufficient pain relief for the doctor to gently scrape clean the cavity of the uterus. This can usually be done by the doctor's fingers, and is a strange experience for the woman who is awake during this procedure, but some women prefer this to a general anaesthetic and if the doctor explains each step of the procedure then it is not too distressing.

When a general anaesthetic is required, the anaesthetist uses an intravenous injection to induce sleep and then puts an endotracheal tube over the back of the tongue and into the windpipe through which pass the gases which keep the woman asleep. This technique is safer than using a mask because in later pregnancy the stomach empties more slowly and so the risk of vomiting under the anaesthetic is greater. Afterwards, it is not uncommon for the woman to complain of a sore throat.

Treatment for an Ectopic Pregnancy

If an ectopic pregnancy is suspected, a laparoscopy is carried out to assess the situation and if an ectopic pregnancy is found the doctors proceed to open up the abdomen – this operation is called a laparotomy. If it is thought that a laparotomy is going to be necessary then it is usual to shave the pubic hair first because the incision in the skin is close to this area and removing the pubic hair reduces the risk of infection. The experience before the operation depends on how acute the situation is. If it is not acute then it is best to wait at least four to six hours from the time the woman last had anything to eat or drink, but if the internal bleeding is severe then the situation is an emergency and the operation needs to go ahead immediately. In this situation it is important to get an intravenous drip up at once to give fluids and blood as soon as possible. The anaesthetist will induce sleep by injecting a drug into the blood stream via the intravenous drip. Then an endotracheal tube is used for the administration of gases during the operation.

The operation of laparoscopy involves looking inside the abdomen with a long thin telescope type instrument. Firstly, a fine hollow needle is inserted into the abdomen just below the navel and some carbon dioxide gas is passed through the needle. The woman is tilted slightly head down, so that the bowel will float upwards towards the diaphragm away from the womb, tubes and ovaries. The telescope type instrument (laparoscope) is then introduced into the abdomen through a small incision made just underneath the navel (about half an inch long) and through this instrument the womb, tubes and ovaries can be viewed and a diagnosis made. If there is no ectopic pregnancy there is usually no need to do anything further and the only scar is the small crescent-shaped scar beneath the navel. If there is an ectopic pregnncy the subsequent treatment will depend on many factors: whether the pregnancy has ruptured through the tube or not; how much bleeding there is; the size of the ectopic pregnancy if unruptured; the site of the ectopic; whether the woman has had a previous ectopic in the same tube or not; whether the woman wants children in the future; whether the tubes were damaged from pre-existing disease; the equipment available and the expertise of the operating surgeon.

Conservative treatment, with preservation of the fallopian tubes may be possible performing a salpingostomy (opening the tube to remove the ectopic but preserving the tube), instead of salpingectomy (removing the tube, plus the ectopic). This can be performed either through the laparoscope or at a laparotomy.

If it has grown close to the end of the tube it is sometimes possible to 'milk' the ectopic pregnancy out of the end of the tube but it is never possible to transfer this tissue to the uterus, which is a question frequently asked before the operation. Unfortunately it is more common to find that the tube has been irrevocably destroyed by the ectopic pregnancy, in which case the tube is removed (salpingectomy). Sometimes, an ectopic pregnancy begins to grow between the end of the tube and the ovary so the ovary will be destroyed as well. When this happens the ovary is also removed but this is uncommon. The remaining ovary will double up to produce the same amount of hormones cyclically each month as two ovaries and ovulation will occur each month from the one ovary. If the ovary on the same side as the affected tube is healthy, it is usually left and ovulation can then occur from either side. It is possible for the tube on the opposite side to the ovary that has just ovulated to pick up the egg.

It is not usually possible to reconstruct a tube either on the affected side or the other side at the same time as operating for an ectopic pregnancy. Non-surgical treatments using Methotrexate, either given to the woman by an intramuscular injection or injected directly into the ectopic pregnancy under ultrasound control are being developed. The pregnancy is destroyed and is gradually reabsorbed by the body. However, it can only be used if the ectopic pregnancy is detected very early on and it is important to keep a close eye on the pregnancy hormone (HCG) levels for several weeks. It is still only a research technique and its use is not widespread.

After a Miscarriage or Ectopic Pregnancy: Physical Changes

After a miscarriage

After a miscarriage bleeding should not be heavier than a period and the colour of the blood loss will change from red to pink or brown. Bleeding will gradually decrease in amount but sometimes continues right up to the first period. If the bleeding gets heavier with blood clots and if there is pain or fever then this could indicate that the uterus is not completely empty or that there is infection. The two problems can go together. If this happens it is important to contact the doctor in case antibiotics are needed to control the infection or a further ERPC is necessary. As explained earlier, it can be difficult for the first ERPC to ensure that the uterus is empty. The average length of stay in hospital for an early miscarriage is between 4 and 6 hours depending on the amount of bleeding, and between 12 and 24 hours for a late miscarriage.

After a late miscarriage there can be the added problem of the breasts producing milk. This can be suppressed with special hormone tablets such as Bromocriptine. Other precautions such as wearing a good supporting bra and pain-killing tablets such as paracetamol may be all that is necessary without using hormones. The important point is not to stimulate the breasts at this time as this will encourage more milk production. The pitfall can be the desire to keep fiddling with the nipples just to see if there is still any milk.

After an ectopic pregnancy

Not only does the woman have to recover from major surgery, and sometimes cope with the awareness that she could have died, but also there is the loss of the pregnancy and probably the loss of part of her body, namely the fallopian tube in which the pregnancy was growing. There may be considerable anxiety about the future and her ability to conceive again with only one tube and her fear of another ectopic pregnancy.

The woman who has had an ectopic pregnancy may need a blood transfusion, and because of all the blood that has been inside her abdomen it may take several days before her bowels start to work so that she can drink and eat again: during that period she will continue to get fluids through a drip. Her stay in hospital will be longer than for a miscarriage, probably about five days, and she will need to convalesce for about a month.

Seeing the Baby

After an early miscarriage there will be little tissue to see and the baby is not usually recognisable, but from about ten weeks onwards the tiny foetus may be recognised, and the further advanced the pregnancy, the more likely this will be. With a later miscarriage the woman may deliver the baby at home and therefore see it, or it may be delivered in the hospital. Most women do want to see the baby, but it helps to discuss the decision with the doctors and nurses. The main thing is for every woman to have the choice of seeing the baby. Not every hospital has a policy of offering this choice when the baby is very small, although the choice is usually offered when the baby is 16 weeks or more.

Seeing and touching the baby can help to answer many questions and remove fear of the unknown. Occasionally the baby may be very deformed and the decision as to whether to see the baby or not is very difficult. Usually the baby can be wrapped in a shawl in such a way as to hide gross deformities and the mother can the decide whether to gradually unwrap and see all of the baby or to keep the memory of the baby wrapped up.

A woman may want to know what has happened to the pregnancy tissue that has come from her womb. Usually, the tissue is sent to the laboratory to confirm that it is pregnancy tissue and to exclude hydatidiform mole. Further tissue may be sent for genetic testing. After these tests the tissue is incinerated. With later miscarriages, the parents may be asked to give consent for a post mortem to be performed on the baby if the doctors feel this could help them find out why the miscarriage occurred and therefore help with counselling about future pregnancies. Tissue may also be sent for genetic testing. Nothing would be done to the baby without the parents' understanding and signed consent and afterwards the body would be incinerated. The parents do have the right to ask for the body to receive a hospital burial or to arrange to take away the body for a private burial.

There are no legal requirements regarding burial except in the following circumstances. Babies born around 22–4 weeks of life may show signs of life by attempting to breathe. Today, it is possible to support some of these very small babies and some will survive. However, the lungs are often too immature and it is not possible to support life for long. The more immature the baby, the less likely are the chances of survival. When there have been signs of life, then the baby will need to have a birth certificate and then a notification of neonatal death certificate. If the baby is born dead after 24 weeks of pregnancy, then a certificate of stillbirth is issued. Legally all babies registered as neonatal deaths or stillbirths must be buried either by the hospital or privately. The hospital admin-istration helps the parents to deal with the necessary certification and to make arrangements for the burial. If the parents choose a burial arranged by the hospital, the baby will be buried in a shared, public grave, rather than in an indidivdually identifiable one, but the hospital or cemetery should be able to indicate the approximate place of burial.

There are no legal requirements regarding burial for infants born dead before 24 weeks – the Home Office gives local authorities the discretion to decide which procedures to adopt. It is worth enquiring what policies are in force locally, as recently at least one local authority has decided to offer a new service to undertake the burial or cremation of babies born dead before 24 weeks of pregnancy (through miscarriage or abortion), provided that a medical practitioner's certification 'in respect of a non-viable foetus' and other relevant forms are completed. This practice will, it is hoped, help the parents to come to terms with their loss more easily and give the baby 'the dignity [in death] of a human being'.[1]

It is usually not possible to see the baby after an ectopic pregnancy. The embryo dies at the time the fallopian tube ruptures and may be expelled with a blood clot into the abdominal cavity or remain within the tube. In either event, it shrivels and is un-recognisable. It also seems that genetic abnormalities are often present in ectopic pregnancies that are related to a failure of the embryo to develop, as described in the section on a 'blighted ovum'. In cases where the embryo is recognisable, it is very small – about 0.5–1.0 cm in length – and usually protected inside a sac inside the tube. It is common for the tissue removed during surgery to be sent to a laboratory to confirm that it is pregnancy tissue within the tube.

Emotional Reactions

After the miscarriage, it is helpful for the couple to have some time alone together and for hospital staff to respect this need for privacy. There is frequently a sense of efficiency in the ward routine which may gloss over the need for privacy and appear to 'sweep under the carpet' the impact of the miscarriage on the couple, or the woman, if she is alone. This doesn't mean that this approach may not be appropriate at the right time. It is also important to give the woman time to talk and express herself: closed questions such as 'You are all right now, aren't you?' may suppress this need. After a miscarriage or ectopic pregnancy a woman may feel numb and unreceptive, so information may well go in one ear and out the other, and so needs to be patiently repeated.

The woman will feel grief, disbelief, anger, 'Why me?', and often guilt – looking for a reason why the miscarriage occurred. She may blame herself, her partner or doctors. If the attack is against another person, it is hard not to take it personally. Speaking from the doctor's point of view, I know I cannot cause a miscarriage by examining a woman internally, but if a woman miscarries soon after I have done so, I can understand that she may link the two events in her mind and it is important not to go on the defensive and alienate the woman if she decides to blame me.

Going home is a difficult time when bottled-up emotions can eventually come to the surface. Perhaps the home has already been prepared for the new baby. Coming home also means facing the family, neighbours, friends, or colleagues at work. Friends and relatives may make unintentionally unkind comments, especially if they are unaware at first that the woman has lost the baby. Commonly, people choose to ignore the fact altogether. These reactions are usually a cover for embarrassment and pain, because it is difficult for others to contemplate the woman's grief. However, there may also be friends and relatives who have experienced a miscarriage, to whom it will be easier to talk and show grief because they have experienced similar suffering. It is often an eyeopener to realise how many friends have had similar experiences but have kept the fact hidden until such time as it can be shared.

If the woman carrying the baby is in a relationship, her partner's feelings also need to be recognised. The partner may have been very frightened at seeing the woman in pain and bleeding and may have feared losing her. There may be feelings of guilt – 'If only we hadn't made love last Friday' – and a man may feel he is a failure – 'Perhaps my sperm wasn't good enough'.

Follow-up Care

The turnover in hospital needs to be fast and some women may interpret this as being cold and unfeeling. However, it is important for all women to have some counselling regarding a future pregnancy and the use of contraception and to have a chance to talk and grieve. Follow up by the hospital team is not possible for most early miscarriages because the volume of work this would create could not be handled. After three (sometimes two) early miscarriages, a woman will be offered further tests and counselling to exclude certain factors for repeated miscarriage. Follow up after later miscarriage (16 weeks or more) is common hospital practice. This usually takes place six weeks later and provides an opportunity for further expression of feelings. The results of the post mortem, blood, genetic and any other tests can be discussed too and further investigations planned if applicable. Counselling about future pregnancies can then be given (see p. 115 on genetic counselling).

Follow up after an ectopic pregnancy will be given by the hospital team about six weeks after the operation. At this visit the scar is checked for healing and further discussion of the reasons for the ectopic pregnancy, feelings about the experience and advice for the future can take place.

Finally, the GP can be a good listener, especially in times of depression that may come unexpectedly some time after the miscarriage, such as at that time when the baby would have been born. A subsequent pregnancy can also be a time of anxiety until the time of an earlier miscarriage has passed and even a successful birth may be tinged with feelings of sadness for the baby that didn't make it.

The Future

Periods

With the bleeding immediately after a miscarriage or ectopic pregnancy, it is important to use pads and not tampons because of the risk of introducing infection to the uterus, but by the time of the first period it is safe to use tampons again. The first period usually comes four to six weeks later and may well be particularly heavy and painful, as if the womb is having its own spring clean. The second period is more likely to be normal.

Contraception

After a miscarriage any form of contraceptive would be satisfactory but if the woman hopes to conceive again in the near future then a barrier method such as the sheath, diaphragm or cap is preferable. If she wishes to wait for several months or years, the combined pill, progesterone-only pill, the coil or longacting progestrogen injections or implants could be considered. The choice will depend on the woman's preference and health. Some women prefer to use the safe period and monitor their own cycles, but it will be at least two months and two periods before they are likely to return to a reliable pattern.

After an ectopic pregnancy it is not advisable to have a coil fitted or to use the progesterone-only pill. Both forms of contraception are linked with an increased risk of ectopic pregnancy. The choice of the right contraceptive and referral back to the GP or to a family planning clinic for further advice may help.

Sexual relationships

It is best to avoid intercourse for at least two weeks after a miscarriage to allow the lining of the womb to heal. If there is bleeding for more than two weeks it is better to avoid intercourse until after the first period. These precautions help to reduce the complication of infection. After an ectopic pregnancy it will take about four to six weeks for the womb to heal so that intercourse can occur without causing pain.

Before full intercourse occurs, however, there is no harm in enjoying all the other aspects of love play that do not involve penetration. It really depends on how the couple feels. It may be that feeling depressed after a miscarriage will lower libido, or perhaps the woman may fear a further pregnancy and therefore fear resuming a sexual relationship. If this occurs then the couple will need to seek further advice and counselling. Perhaps just reliable contraception or reassurance about future pregnancies is all that is necessary, but sometimes other problems may be brought to the surface by the miscarriage and need deeper counselling.

Masturbation after a miscarriage is safe and orgasm can help with 'clearing' out any small pieces of tissue still inside the womb. However, after an ectopic pregnancy an orgasm is likely to be painful for the first four weeks and experiencing pain could be frightening and lead to emotional problems later when resuming a sex life with a partner.

Work and leisure

After a miscarriage the woman may need from a couple of days up to a week of resting to recover physically and also to get stronger emotionally before returning to work (both paid employment and work in the home). Some women like to get back to work quickly and lose themselves in keeping busy, others feel the need for a period of peace and quiet before facing the outside world again. After an ectopic pregnancy the woman will need about a month off work to convalesce. Hopefully, relatives and friends will be able to help.

As far as leisure activities are concerned, it is best to listen to your own body and do what you feel capable of doing. It is best to avoid swimming in public baths for the first two weeks as this could be a source of infection.

Future pregnancies

After a miscarriage I usually advise a woman to wait for two periods before trying for a further pregnancy. This gives the woman's hormones time to settle down into a regular cycle and gives some time for emotional healing. It may be very hard to wait longer, but there is evidence that the risk of a further miscarriage is greater if the woman conceives in the first cycle after a miscarriage. Waiting until after the second period has the added advantage of making it easier to date the next pregnancy. I usually advise that after an ectopic pregnancy the woman should wait for three periods before trying again. This gives her plenty of time to heal inside.

The Future for the Medical Profession

So where to do we go in the future? Every gynaecology department needs to look at the way it is handling the problems of miscarriage and other pregnancy losses. For instance, the number of vaginal examinations performed by different doctors should be thought about sympathetically and reduced to the minimum necessary to help elucidate the situation, at the same time appreciating that junior doctors are in a learning situation and will need to have their examination findings checked from time to time. The needs of women and the needs of staff should be constantly reviewed.

From 1994 many gynaecology services are setting up early pregnancy units. These units encourage self-refferal and quicker referral for confirmation of pregnancy or a diagnosis of any early pregnancy problems. This has the advantage that fewer doctors are involved and the woman can be seen more quickly with access to a quick Beta HCG pregnancy test and ultrasound scan for confirmation of any possible problems.

The misunderstandings that arise by the use of the term spontaneous abortion referring to a miscarriage and not a termination of pregnancy should be looked at carefully. Junior nurses or medical students also require thorough education about medical terminology in this field when they come to work on a gynaecology ward so that they do not make the mistake of thinking that a woman having a spontaneous abortion had in some way wanted to lose the baby. The sorrows often experienced by women having an elective abortion also need to be pointed out. Medical training would benefit from focusing more on basic social and counselling skills, rather than the current steady progression towards personnel becoming technological problem-solvers and away from being caring professionals.

The staff working on gynaecology and obstetric wards, both doctors and nurses, would also benefit from discussion and support groups to help them cope with their own feelings of failure and inadequacy in dealing with miscarriage and other pregnancy losses and also to act as a constant reminder to treat every woman as an individual.

The gynaecological location of hospital beds for women experiencing a miscarriage is a difficult topic, which needs to be reviewed by each hospital. Those of us involved in writing this book differed in our opinions. Some felt that women with infertility problems and miscarriage should be kept apart from women coming in for abortions, but others felt that such segregation was false. Many women having abortions also feel sadness because under different personal circumstances they would have wanted the pregnancy to continue and so envy can work both ways. The reality of miscarriage, infertility and abortion as being part of womankind's experience may be better dealt with by keeping women together. If the groups are separated, this may be preferable provided that one group is not obviously 'ostracised'.

We are all part of society and a large part of progress in the future must lie with the ability to change. Women still need to be freed from their subservient role. Education in schools and in the home should aim to prepare all children to take responsibility for their sexuality. We need better education about contraception, pregnancy and childbirth and a more realistic approach to the problems of pregnancy and parenthood. The aspect of 'failure' needs the same attention as 'success' and should be brought out of the shadows.

Reproductive Resources: Genetic Counselling, Diagnostic Technology and Late Termination of Pregnancy

Fran Reader

Revised by Fran Reader
and Kirsten Duckitt

Genetic Counselling

A genetic counsellor is usually a doctor who specialises in advising a couple about the likelihood of a genetic problem occurring in future babies. The couple may wish to know about the risks because of a strong family history of inherited disorders or recurrent miscarriages, or perhaps they may have already given birth to a child with problems and they would like to know the risk of the problem occurring in a subsequent child.

First, the genetic counsellor will take details of the health of the close family from both partners, and may take blood samples from the couple themselves, to see if they are carriers for any inherited disorders. If blood tests are involved, it takes about three weeks before an answer can be given. Usually the genetic counsellor is able to give the couple some idea of the risks involved at once, but this is not always possible. Some other screening techniques are discussed below.

Ultrasound scan

This helps the doctor to see whether the developing baby appears to be normal. Early in pregnancy the woman is asked to drink plenty of fluids before the scan so that her bladder is full in order to push the womb up higher and make it easier to see. Later in pregnancy an empty bladder may be preferred. In early pregnancy it is common to perform the ultrasound scans vaginally. This means that the transducer part of the machine is gently inserted into the woman's vagina to enable the information coming from the womb to be picked up and displayed on the scan machine. The size of the transducer head for transvaginal scans is roughly equivalent to the size of a small tube of Smarties. Alternatively the scan can be performed through the abdominal wall. In this situation the woman's abdomen is greased and the transducer head used to pass over the abdomen is roughly the size and shape of an audio-cassette'. High frequency sound waves are beamed from this machine on to the uterus and the pattern of the sound is recorded on video as the sound waves bounce off the baby and the placenta. The video picture is rather blurred and needs skilled interpretation, but it can date a pregnancy quite accurately, detect a multiple pregnancy or abnormalities in the shape of the uterus and show the position of the placenta. Ultrasound cannot show up all foetal abnormalities but will help to detect major physical abnormalities that could be life threatening.

Screening for spina bifida, anencephaly and Down's syndrome – the triple test

The triple test is also known as triple screening, maternal serum screening for Down's syndrome, or occasionally as the Bart's test due to it originally being developed at St Bartholomew's Hospital. It is a blood test performed between 15 and 20 weeks of pregnancy (ideally at 16 weeks) which helps identify pregnancies which are at risk of Down's syndrome or other abnormalities such as neural tube defects (e.g. spina bifida and anencephaly). It does this by measuring the amounts of three substances (some hospitals may do a double test that just measures two substances). The three substances are called alpha feto protein (AFP), human chorionic gonadotrophin (HCG) and unconjugated oestriol (UE3) in the mother's blood. Down's syndrome pregnancies are connected with a lower amount of AFP and UE3 and a raised amount of HCG than normal. These measurements along with maternal age and the gestation of the pregnancy as calculated by ultrasound are used to calculate a risk factor for Down's syndrome. It cannot definitely say whether the baby has Down's syndrome or not. It can only produce a risk estimate. If the risk is greater than 1 in 250 (1 in 200 in some hospitals) the mother is offered an amniocentesis, to confirm definitely whether the baby has Down's syndrome or not.

If the risk is lower than 1 in 250 no further action is taken although this does not absolutely rule out the fact that the baby may have Down's syndrome. If the AFP is raised while the other levels remain normal, this may suggest a neural tube defect or other structural abnormality of the baby. A detailed ultrasound scan is then carried out to look carefully at the brain, the spine and other structure.

Down's syndrome babies are more frequently born to women who are older. A woman of 40 has a 1 in 100 risk of a Down's syndrome baby. The incidence of neural tube defects is not related to the mother's age. It occurs as frequently as 1 in 300 pregnancies in some regions of the British Isles, especially in the west.

The Harris Scan

The Harris Scan is a special transabdominal ultrasound scan taken at 11 weeks as a screening test for Down's syndrome. It can be used as an alternative to the triple screen or as a back-up. An area of the back of the foetal skull known as the nuchal fold is measured for thickness. If this area is thicker than 3mm there is a high chance of chromosomal abnormalities, particularly Down's syndrome.

Screening for blood disorders

Some families have certain hereditary blood disorders which can affect children, for example, haemophilia, which is a disorder of blood clotting, or thalasaemia, which is a severe form of anaemia that is particularly a problem amongst families from Greece. Turkey and other Mediterranean countries. These hereditary blood disorders and other eventually fatal conditions such as muscular dystrophy can be diagnosed by chorionic villus sampling (CVS).

Diagnostic Technology

Amniocentesis

Amniocentesis is usually offered to women where the triple test has indicated a risk of Down's syndrome greater than 1 in 250. Some hospitals still offer women over 35 amniocentesis for Down's syndrome regardless of the result of the triple screen. This test is carried out between 16 and 17 weeks of pregnancy and involves taking some of the fluid from around the baby. The doctor checks the position of the baby and the placenta with an ultrasound scan machine, locates a pool of liquor (water around the baby) and marks the mother's skin overlying the pool. This area of skin is then cleansed and a small local anaesthetic injection may be given into the skin to make it numb. Then a fine needle is pushed through the skin and muscle of the womb into this pool of liquor and some of the fluid is removed using a syringe. Cells shed into liquor from the baby's skin can then be isolated and cultured. The genetic make-up of the cells can be examined.

It takes about three weeks to obtain an answer to this test. If there is a genetic abnormality then the mother will be offered a termination of pregnancy. By this time she will be 19 or 20 weeks pregnant. Rarely, the cells isolated may not grow the first time, so the amniocentesis may need to be repeated which brings the time of possible termination later into the pregnancy. The time waiting for an answer and all the uncertainty can be very stressful. Rapid karyotyping at any time in pregnancy is now becoming available and is typically offered if the first culture fails. The rate of miscarriage following the amniocentesis is approximately 1 in 200.

The amniocentesis may be difficult if the placenta is on the front wall of the uterus or if there are fibroids on the front wall, so occasionally the test is not technically feasible.

Cordocentesis

Cordocentesis is a technique used to sample foetal blood in the mid-trimester when interuterine infection is suspected or to check the haemoglobin when the foetus is affected by rhesus disease. Ultrasound is used to locate the place where the umbilical cord is inserted into the placenta. A fine needle is then passed through the uterus to this site under ultrasound control and blood is sampled.

The rate of miscarriage following cordocentesis is approximately 1 in 50 to 1 in 100.

Chorionic villus sampling

This is a technique that has been developed to assist in making the antenatal diagnosis of an abnormality in the first trimester of pregnancy. If an abnormality is confirmed, an abortion can be offered at a stage that is physically safer for the woman and perhaps more emotionally acceptable. There are now hospitals in most of the health regions of Great Britain which are developing skills in chorionic villus sampling (CVS). Women can be referred from their own district hospital to a specialised unit for the test and then return to their own district to continue the pregnancy if all is well.

The technique involves taking a very small sample of early placental tissue containing chorionic villi. These are small microscopic finger-like projections in the placental tissue that carry blood from the developing embryo into close proximity with the mother's blood circulating in the womb, so that transfer of food to, and waste products from, the embryo can occur. The DNA in the genetic material isolated from this tissue is tested. The time taken to obtain a result is between a few days and two weeks, depending on the actual test required.

The sampling is achieved under ultrasound control either by passing a fine plastic tube through the cervix to the region of the developing placenta or by using a fine needle to reach the same tissue through the woman's lower abdomen. The test is usually performed around nine or ten weeks of pregnancy and does carry a risk of miscarriage of around five cases in 100. This risk is lessening with the development of new techniques and medical expertise. Also it must be remembered that at nine to ten weeks of pregnancy a certain number of pregnancies would be expected to miscarry naturally.

Late Termination of Pregnancy

Late terminations of pregnancy are offered when an abnormality is discovered. The woman may then be anything from 17 to 24 weeks pregnant.

The use of prostaglandin

The methods of termination of pregnancy at this stage usually involves a hormone known as prostaglandin, which causes contractions of the muscle of the uterus which will precipitate a miscarriage. Prostaglandin is delivered via a vaginal pessary inserted close to the cervix every three hours. Alternatively the prostaglandin can be injected via a small catheter placed through the cervix so that small increments of the hormone can be given at regular intervals. Both techniques bring on contractions of the uterus which open up the cervix leading to a miscarriage. Prostaglandins can also be given via a drip or injected directly into the amniotic fluid by a technique similar to amniocentesis. Some hospitals use a combination of methods but all have the same outcome. The length of time it takes for the induced miscarriages to occur is very variable – from about six hours up to two days, or occasionally even longer. The pain of the contractions can be helped by strong pain-killing injections or by a drip delivering intravenous pain-killers. The woman can be in control of the rate of the drip within pre-set limits. This is called patient-controlled analgesia (PCA). Finally, pain relief can be achieved by the use of an epidural.

Some hospitals now use the drug RU486, 48 hours before the insertion of prostaglandin pessaries. The RU486 affects the hormone control of the pregnancy and is likely to reduce the time interval between commencing the use of prostaglandins and delivery of the foetus. In later pregnancy some units will use potassium chloride injected under ultrasound control in the foetal heart. This will kill the foetus. These techniques may be considered more humane in the situation where the foetus is grossly abnormal but may well show signs of life for a few minutes which can be distressing for the woman, her partner and her carers.

Once the foetus has been delivered, the placenta may come away as well but sometimes it is retained inside the uterus and needs to be removed. This can be done using an epidural for pain relief or a general anaesthetic can be given.

Dilatation and evacuation (D and E)

Some doctors prefer to peform late terminations of pregnancy by a method known as dilatation and evacuation. In the hands of a doctor experienced in this technique it may be a safer method for the woman than prostaglandin termination. However, not many doctors in this country have the necessary skills.

Before the operation a prostaglandin pessary is inserted into the vagina to soften and open the cervix. The termination itself is performed under a general anaesthetic so the woman is asleep and does not 'experience' the termination. The cervix will have become soft and partially open in response to the pessary but the doctor may need to stretch it open a little more with dilators. Through the open cervix the doctor can pass instruments into the uterus which will remove the foetus and the placenta in bits and pieces. It is therefore not possible to see the whole foetus after such a procedure.

Decision making

I would like to look in more depth at the problems of genetic counselling and antenatal diagnosis. For everyone involved there will be strong emotional, ethical and perhaps religious dilemmas to face. A healthy baby is very much desired but the woman may feel unable to cope with a severely disabled child, mentally or physically, and also feel that the suffering to the child itself would be wrong. However, the actual decision to end the pregnancy can be very difficult to make. Of the tests described, ultrasound and blood tests carry no risk to the developing child; but both amniocentesis and cordocentesis do carry a risk to the baby of possible miscarriage, infection or later of premature delivery. For amniocentesis, the risks of complications are in the order of one in 200 but for fetoscopy the risk is higher at around three in 100. These values vary from centre to centre and the procedures are getting safer as technology and techniques improve. However, it is possible that after a test which shows that the baby is normal the woman may then go on to miscarry or deliver prematurely and the baby not survive. This is naturally a very distressing experience and very hard for the couple to come to terms with. However much the woman may have listened to the risks when counselled beforehand, she will always have hoped it could never happen to her.

If the tests show that the baby is affected, a decision has to be made whether or not to terminate the pregnancy. This is very difficult, as such pregnancies are usually planned and a healthy baby really wanted and expected. Also by the time decisions have to be made, the baby's movements may have been felt by the mother. There may be many emotions involved in reaching a decision: grief, disappointment at 'why me?', fear of the procedure itself, fear that there may be no further pregnancies or that the same thing could happen again, and guilt.

It can be helpful to see the baby after an induced miscarriage. Not everyone feels ready to face this immediately after the delivery, but some may wish to see the baby before leaving the hospital. This experience can help them to come to terms with their decision and helps with subsequent grieving. Other people do not feel able to see the baby; it is easier for them not to have such memories. When the method used for later termination has been a D and E it will not be possible to see the baby and this needs to be thought about beforehand. In this situation some symbolic burial act may help grieving (see Part Four).

I have tended to refer to couples in this situation but a woman may be alone in having to make these difficult decisions and to experience the termination on her own. Even in a strong supportive relationship the woman may still feel very alone at this time, as the emotions felt by both partners (whether male or female) are very deep and can be hard to express, especially those of anger and guilt. But, however difficult it may be to express feelings, it helps to talk and to share the feelings and allow emotions to show.

Many hospitals are now becoming better equipped to deal with late termination of pregnancy for foetal abnormality. Some hospitals have special suites for women undergoing induced labour in these circumstances. Both doctors and midwives receive more training in how to support the woman and her partner through the experience.

Part Three:
The Key Issues:
Making Sense of Our Stories

A Feminist Exploration

Valerie Hey

Introduction

This chapter aims to provide a narrative framework enabling the reader to place and understand the 'inside stories' which precede it. Although written by one woman, it could not have been written in its current form without the benefit of sharing our biographies and working together for an analysis. This way of working and sharing owes an enormous debt to the women's movement, which is the context to our own lives and which was for us the initial and continuing resource for our friendships, ideas and political practices. This opening analysis aims to show and share the fruits of the difficult but rewarding process of collective endeavour.

It does not claim to supply all of the answers. Neither is it presented as a set of statements about how one *should* feel. We want to get away totally from such prescriptions. Thus whilst it is a record of our encounters with 'a different sort of death', as one of us called miscarriage and ectopic pregnancy, it is offered in the full acknowledgement that what for us was a problem, for other women might be a solution. We go on to try and translate this recognition into a new and more fully expressed politics of reproduction later, but this chapter tries to account for how *we* felt and to link that understanding to our experiences of being female in a society which is male-dominated. As such it may offer the reader a way into explaining her own inside story, or it may, as I've noted, raise points of difference between her experience and the experiences described here.

Indeed, no two of us reacted identically. We each managed our experiences in unique ways; some of us were still in shock months after, whilst others expressed their distress as very much the heart of the actual physical process. But just as importantly, there were common reactions. We became aware of this common ground as we explored together the meanings we made of our individual biographies. Themes emerged from our exchanges about our feelings and our management in hospitals which gradually began to clarify the personal as *the political*. Had this not occurred, the ensuing overview would not have materialised. Its existence records our struggles to come to terms personally and politically with our hidden loss as feminists, just as much as the chapters detailing the more explicitly therapeutic strategies.

An important feature of this collective enterprise is that it challenges both the forms of our oppression and our uncritical acceptance of aspects of its work. Thus this coming to terms has not been an altogether comfortable journey. We, too, have had to recognise our own resentment of other women for whom pregnancy is straightforward, just as we have had to acknowledge a need to embrace those women who have chosen abortion. Some of us were initially resistant to those ideas. Then we began to see that this resistance stemmed from a socially constructed division between women, one which is usually perceived as natural. This makes some women – those who miscarry – worthy of compassion, and others – those who have a termination – deserving of blame. These competitive relations are constructed from the *identical* polarities of innocence and guilt which form one of the major organising principles of patriarchal control. (This can also be seen in the different kinds of treatment meted out to women who have been raped, according to how much 'to blame' they are for the assault.)

Our attitudes have *had* to move, especially since some of us have had both abortions and miscarriages or ectopic pregnancies. This book is premised on these shifts – it is based on a fundamental recognition that we could not reconcile ourselves *with the old terms*.

As the Preface to the book made clear, this book represents a new contribution to the politics of women's health and to the wider and more contentious and indivisible issue of reproductive rights. It is with the making of a new language in new terms that this analysis is primarily concerned.

Important themes in the chapter include:

1

Paradoxes of prebirth or birth loss. This latter term is possibly more meaningful here since a number of the contributors to this book describe their miscarriage as resembling the birthing experience.

2

Aspects of analysis. This looks at the management of our birth loss by the medical establishment as an exercise in power. More particularly it elaborates a process through which female experience is 'handled' so as to all but silence its complexity and intensity. We did not receive understanding; instead we witnessed the partial nature of science and the privileging of 'facts'. This section examines one of the most obvious means by which the suppression of 'inadmissible' evidence is achieved – by focusing upon language in considerable detail we try to elaborate the alienating dynamics of our medical encounters.

Throughout the chapter it is argued that male 'expertise' contributes more significantly to our pain than to its alleviation.

Paradoxes of Pregnancy and Prebirth Loss

The literature, the cultural messages we receive, our mothers, and shared collective common sense make it seem that having a baby as the result of being pregnant is as automatically guaranteed as rain in June.

There are good reasons why this is the case, linked to the way femininity in our culture is defined in the language of marriage, domesticity and child-rearing (preferably in that order!). Motherhood as the natural consequence of wifehood is the socially approved female destiny. Examination of the social structures, customs and controls making this the case is not the main purpose of this account. But a recognition of the primacy of marriage and children in adult lives must necessarily provide the ideological and social frame for any consideration of our particular negative maternal experiences.

Marriage and the status that being a wife bestows has other attractions that we should not forget. Monogamous heterosexuality remains the only socially acceptable form for the expression of sexuality. For young women, marriage is one of the major means through which they achieve recognition as mature adults.

At another level, the importance of motherhood for us also reflects upon unconscious desires for access to babyhood and childhood, as unique and valuable parts of experience which we can re-enter in another form through our children. I find this aspect of parenthood a rich but neglected area for discussion. Certainly my own pleasures in my daughters' childhood are enhanced through the empathies they arouse in me. In the light of children's relative powerlessness this insight could form the basis of new understandings about parent/carer and child relationships which offer a way of dealing with the complex feelings we have as our children's powerful others. This is an identity which so often contradicts our sense of ourselves as victims both of our children and of circumstances outside our control.

To return to the focus of my argument, I am saying that the seductiveness of motherhood is no more an obvious effect of conditioning than it is of our nature: the multidimensional desire for it makes its possibility or impossibility such a powerful determinant in our lives.

Even if you decide irrevocably *against* it, it is still a force to be reckoned with. After all, the womb is one of our biggest physical differences from men and its processes, potentialities and particularities measure out our lives in quite distinct ways.

Thus the underpinning of maternity by physical, cultural and ideological factors ensures its centrality in female lives. This is the context in which we all conceived. We held what now appears an over-optimistic, not to say naïve view that birth follows pregnancy as sure as night follows day. We were pregnant, we were expecting a baby. We had no reason to expect that it would be otherwise.

Whilst we had no reason to think that our pregnancies would 'fail' the context for women experiencing pregnancy loss today is more complicated. Paradoxically women in Western societies may find themselves, in the context of newer technologies of pre-conception and prebirth diagnostic and surveillance techniques, even more distressed by unpredictable outcomes, in what has become a highly technocratic regime of maternal care. The introduction of a battery of tests actually seems to promise certainties but the experiential reality reveals that these techniques (e.g. chorionic villus sampling) do not guarantee immunity from miscarriage. Arguments mobilised by feminists about the need for women to control the terms of birth have extended the choices available more positively in women's favour, and these will be discussed later. Nevertheless it is important to recognise that although the combined and contradictory impact of such extensions of 'choice' fundamentally change expectations about maternity, they do not displace the feelings of shock when pregnancies deviate from the 'normal'. The present highly technicist forms of monitoring merely make the scope of the ethical and emotional dilemmas which women have to confront more complex, as they seek to make sense of a particular rupture at the heart of the maternity experience.

There can be no accurate data on pregnancies which are lost, since some women lose pregnancies before they realise they are pregnant. Considering the fact that *at least* one in five pregnancies fails, it is bizarre that such information and such a common experience remains hidden: maternity's best-kept secret.

Our ignorance is made possible by the general taboo in Western society about speaking of death, a silence which, added to the secrecy surrounding 'women's troubles' and the need to maintain the ideology of blissful motherhood, produces the comprehensive evasions surrounding the experiences of miscarriage and ectopic pregnancy.

In searching for details to confirm or explain our stories, we have to look hard to find our experiences represented. We appear, if at all, as the footnotes in the pregnancy literature, filed away under the abnormal. Even ectopic pregnancy, which is a relatively rare form of prebirth loss, happens one in 300 conceptions. Moreover if 20 per cent of conceptions are abnormal, it should then be recognised that these experiences require more acknowledgement than cursory allusions tacked on to the main text of maternity literature.

One of the results of these self-cancelling messages is perplexing confusion. On the one hand we are told to 'remember the right to life of an unborn child' if we seek an abortion. Yet on the other hand, if we do not elect to terminate our child's life but we miscarry or 'abort spontaneously', we are expected to act *as if we were never pregnant*. We are told, 'Oh, you were only x weeks pregnant,' and encouraged to 'pull yourself together', to 'try again', and to 'be thankful for your existing children' (if we have any). We may be told it was 'God's will' or, more tactlessly still, that it was 'a blessing in disguise; the baby would have been deformed'.

If being pregnant is considered the epitome of femininity, assuming we have the right status – married; are the right age – 25–30; are the right colour and class – white, upwardly mobile and thus demonstrably responsible in every regard, then being un-pregnant after a miscarriage or ectopic pregnancy is like being in limbo, where we are supposed to act as if our 'little bit of a problem' is too trivial to talk about. This sense of our abandonment alerts us to the deeper meanings which our experience poses for those with whom we come into contact.

One way into unravelling the paradox is to begin with the material event: as a physical occurrence a death before a birth is itself the ultimate paradox. We are at one moment nurturing life and the next minute embracing death, and at times the distinction cannot be clearly made, as Janet's reactions remind us:

And I had been shown my baby, still inside me. S/he had been measured and given an age. And I had shown detached interest in the wonders of technology. And it was the depth of my despair, the loudest of my silent screaming, the most desolate loneliness. All inadmissible. And if this baby had died, it had not also left me. 'But we cannot be absolutely certain that it is not alive. So let's leave it for a while, see what happens, look again.' Six days of not knowing whether I was carrying life or death inside me.

In the very enclosure which ought to guarantee safety we are harbouring a dead baby, and just as in stillbirth, those women who have late miscarriages undergo a labour process with the knowledge that there will be no happy outcome. This consciousness of irredeemable pain is prevalent in all of the personal accounts, and is just as true of early as of late miscarriage.

Most of us who were admitted to hospital as a consequence of our ectopic pregnancy/miscarriage found ourselves in a strange country, with professionals who spoke a different dialect.

Alice Lovell quotes from the experience of other women:

A woman whose pregnancy does not result in the usual happy event presents embarrassing problems. There is no live baby to join the other squalling bundles in the nursery, and the woman no longer qualifies as a mother – even if she has other children at home. She and her baby are misfits. The solution to this dilemma lies in disposing of the evidence as quickly as possible. After a 'rugger pass' to get rid of the baby, the mother has to be disposed of too. Usually she is put into a room by herself and sent home as fast as possible.[1]

This awkwardness is registered by most of us, and it took many forms, with many consequences. It is one of the frameworks within which to place our accounts, as if to hold on to the validity of our emotions we had to fight back against the embarrassment we were causing. As one of Alice Lovell's respondents said so powerfully, 'I had a pregnancy, but then I was thrown out of the club'.

Being thrown out of the club is very much written into the pregnancy narrative anyway, as many mothers know. Once you've been successfully delivered you are on your own, sister! The antenatal concern which centres upon the state of your body, your diet, your habits and your life-style abruptly ceases once you enter the postnatal phase. The aftercare consists principally of tactless contraceptive advice and a postnatal examination presumptuously geared to checking out your continuing availablity for penetrative and hence normative heterosexuality.[2]

However, if you become a mother you enter the other club, as many women have noted – the secret club of maternity where along with other mums you swop inside information and knowing looks. But being unpregnant leaves you apparently with no clubs left to join. You are thus cut off from the sort of support you need. Forced to 'suffer in silence' initially, most of us did not continue this self-betrayal. Sooner or later we began to search out the hidden knowledge which is not public but which exists in fragmented and privatised forms in individual women's memories and lives.

If you are lucky, they too will admit their own miscarriages, their own hidden losses, and in so doing help you to stop feeling alone and misunderstood. Of all the early contacts I had with women after my own miscarriage, it was a telephone conversation I had with my aunt (who had lost a baby at nearly full term in the 1940s) which made the most sense to me. Far more than the injunctions to 'get over it' or the other conventional platitudes which we utter in the face of difficult experiences, her words to me, born out of shared sorrow, touched the truth of my own feelings – confirming my right to them.

Turning in more detail to our accounts, I particularly want to ask why our versions of events are silenced within popular and professional discourse. I want to begin this critical investigation by looking at aspects of the nature of hospital culture, since this was for most or all of us the single most provocative encounter – where we came up against the alienating professional codes and routines that resulted in us feeling worse rather than better.

Aspects of an Analysis: Hierarchies of Knowledge or Just What The Doctor Ordered!

Recent shifts to the introduction of what Le Grand calls 'quasi-markets' in the Health Service have opened up spaces within hospital settings for the introduction of regimens of care which might be said to be more 'customer-friendly'. Certainly there has been an uneven collision inside the Health Service between feminist ideas and the market principle. Hospitals now commission 'needs assessments' seeking to quantify the sort of services which their 'customers' want. It is important to locate the shift to home births and more nuanced maternity services (the availability of active births, the use of outside alternative birth preparation courses) as responses to both types of differently inspired interventions. Nevertheless hospitals, like so many other institutions, reflect the distribution of power in wider society. Walk into most reception areas and the general pattern will be of white male doctors, black female domestics. The status of male authority is literally acted out around each bed during every consultant's round, when the (usually white) god descends with his acolytes. The day-to-day essential nursing by women is more and more undervalued as government priorities pay lip service to the 'angels' only to continue to underpay them. It is male heroic medicine which grabs both the cash and the headlines.

Unsurprisingly, when women enter hospital they find that these institutions have their own rationales, 'they do things differently there'. As Lesley noted in a letter to Mary Anne, only in a hospital would you get woken up to be given a sleeping pill!

This culture's particular deference to medicine as both a practice and a profession gives male expertise even more hallowed status than usual. This arises partly as a result of the primacy of the scientific medical model within the NHS and partly from the relations of dependency we are forced into as part of the 'being-ill script'. If we are continually encouraged to defer to authority in general and male authority in particular, and if we are placed in these subordinate relations when also frightened and in pain, we are multiply disadvantaged and it is very difficult to express a right to being treated seriously in all senses of the word.

Our self-understandings are merely reduced to information for the endless forms that have to be filled in. Few professionals have the sense to listen to us, the time which good-quality listening takes, or the humanity and confidence to admit that they are not always able to give us definitive answers.

In researching for this book I came across one particularly startling example of these processes, where a woman's account of her pregnant status was totally discredited by both her husband and the health-care professionals who were overseeing her case. She had been expecting twins but miscarried and yet she still felt herself to be definitely pregnant, with the signs of vomiting and fatigue. No one believed her. They told her it was a phantom pregnancy and that she was 'imagining it'. Her insistence so disturbed her husband and her doctor that they colluded in obtaining her admission to a psychiatric ward. Eventually she began to *show* her pregnancy and the one baby who had survived the miscarriage of its twin was found via an ultrasound scan.[4]

Mary Anne describes a less dramatic instance of her knowledge about her body being discounted:

I was finally put in a cubicle, on a couch and waited for the doctor. He finally came and we went through all the questions again: why am I here; what are my dates. 'Oh, well, it's a bit early for a first visit.' 'Yes, but I've been bleeding and I've got these pains in my side. My GP thought it best to check . . .' 'Oh . . . Do you want to be pregnant?' 'Yes, I do.' (And it's not a phantom pregnancy, which I can see you think it is; it's not all in my imagination – it's real, I've had other signs.) 'We don't have a positive urine test.' 'But you can't be sure; my breasts are tender and bigger; my sleep pattern's changed,' etc. etc. Silently, 'Why don't you listen to me, to what my body is saying?'

Integral to this process of devaluation is the tension created by the interpretation of our inside stories through the language of outsiders. The principal way in which we felt excluded from the business of getting our needs met was the reduction of our complex experiences to a purely medical/physical event. I will go on to show this in practice by looking at the dominant language of health-care professionals. I argue that what it represses is as interesting as what it expresses.

The Language of Control

Earlier I mentioned the paradoxical nature of the physical facts of a death-birth/prebirth loss. From the 'inside stories' you may recall both Ann and Valerie actually feeling as if they *had given birth*; I expressed it in the cryptic phrase 'I felt as if I'd achieved something'. This, I now realise, was primarily made from the feeling and experience of birthing, despite my low-key manner at the time of acting brave and calm, of complying outwardly with the management of it as a miscarriage. Janet's account too, speaks of this dissonance between the inner turmoil and the outer surface of control – of 'being sensible' whilst also wanting to say, 'Keep the baby, don't throw it down the sluice. I want to see it.'

For all of us, the meaning of our experiences was indivisible from the emotions provoked by the physical events. I had read that I was having a 'late miscarriage' but I felt at the end as if I had given birth.

The fact is that, unavoidably, we experience the physical side of the ectopic pregnancy or miscarriage alone. Recognising that aloneness without trying to deny it is a prerequisite for being supportive to a woman who is losing a baby. Janet expresses this separation at the heart of her experience as central to her sense of emotional distress:

> We had always been together. We had believed that pregnancy, labour, delivery was *our* experience, not just mine. But the physical experience could not be shared, and it is the physical experience that reminds you, every minute, every second . . . It doesn't leave you alone. 'Pure' feelings of grief and fear became contaminated with 'nasty' feelings of resentment and anger and frustration in being unable to communicate, and disappointment that, after all, I did not have the unity I thought I had.

In this sense therefore we are on our own. But the chief part of my argument is that if this is the isolating reality (how we feel about it is often represented in our stories as concern at literally not being left alone), then how we are handled, both in language and in others' actions, becomes of crucial concern. We have no knowledge to warn us of what to expect, no guidance as to what to do. Sheila, normally used to taking responsibility for herself and others, could not cope with the prospect of the threatened loss of her child as described in *Our Bodies, Ourselves*: 'The foetus, amniotic sac and placenta . . . may be expelled completely intact.[5] The answer she gives to why this description made her desperate to get to hospital before *it* finally happened was that she 'just could not comprehend the thought of actually producing a partially developed foetus – our future baby.'

A major problem with the authorised/medicalised versions is, most obviously and immediately, their alienating language. Sheila's incapacity to cope registers in part the alienation which we all felt from the medical vocabulary. Talk of 'foetus', 'products of conception' or even more perplexingly of 'spontaneous abortion' simply could not be reconciled with our feelings of conceiving and wanting a baby. We had not been expecting a 'foetus'. We had not anticipated a 'product of conception' joining our household. Within one short phrase Sheila is in struggle to name her appropriate reality. Whilst foetus is the correct medical term, using it depersonalises the experience – to keep those threatening emotions *and* the professionals under control.

Recognising this loss as our future baby moves it to another, more demanding frame of reference both for ourselves and for those who care for us. It is explicitly about accepting the two inseparable elements in prebirth loss, namely the physical *and* the emotional. Health-care professionals are understandably more responsive to the routines of managing and monitoring the physical side of reproductive medicine, if only because the predominant form of National Health Service care is modelled on reactive/interventionist medicine.

Actually this model also provides insights into why miscarriage is so mismanaged. Miscarriage is an under-researched area, unpopular because it seems intractably resistant to solution, and interventionism has spectacularly failed to prevent its occurrence. (Intervention in the case of ectopic pregnancy, on the other hand, is essential and life-saving – yet the fact that a baby is being lost gets forgotten in the medical drama of emergency surgery.) The failure of effective intervention in the case of miscarriage, I believe, contributes to the response of health workers, who treat the event casually so as to make their ineffectiveness less problematic. Another way that workers are able to distance themselves from women is to treat the situation purely as a matter of routine – a tendency greatly exacerbated by the underfunding of NHS provision.

This reductive management of prebirth loss – through avoidance or procedural and routine – is also related to the very nature of hospital life, in which workers are having to deal with life and death as part of their daily workload. Indeed, as many of us found (though it was no comfort at the time!) prebirth loss *is* common. As Janet says in response to this: 'Common to him, but not to me.'

One gets a sense that this safe language works primarily as self-protection for professionals whose daily life is made up of so many potentially emotionally charged dramas. However, holding on to the certainties of scientific terminology is all the more ironic in a situation where science has so little to offer by way of explanation of the causes and management of threatened prebirth loss. It frequently seemed that the less health professionals could provide answers to our questions of why, how, what about the future, the more the medical framework was applied. It is almost as if the rationale for its continued use needed to be *re*-asserted in the face of the ambiguities, uncertainties and contradictions of losing a baby before term; as if our failure had to be neatly tidied up so that the threatened fuss would not spill out and draw attention to the medical profession's failure too.

My concentration upon the politics of language is not merely a question of raising awareness about the need for sensitivity for its own sake. I want to suggest that giving us the right to claim the experience in our own words makes us better able to begin the process of recovery. We found from our own experiences that in the short term we were misunderstood and marginalised, and in the longer term actively hindered in the business of getting better by the conspiracy of silence which followed being in that post-birth-but-no-baby limbo.

Even within its *own* terms I want to claim the medical model as hopelessly inadequate with respect to the actual physical account of miscarriage or ectopic pregnancy. It is instructive to explore the distortion of our experiences in the language used to describe the likely course of a miscarriage – which, we were told time and time again, was likely to involve 'slight cramping' at least or resemble a 'heavy period' at most. Notice that the model against which the experience is measured is that of menstruation rather than labour. This is highly significant, I think, and is linked to the whole way in which the loss is medicalised and managed. By comparing our pain to that of the humdrum business of monthly blood loss (and this is what doctors are taught!), the child metaphorically disappears, the emotional temperature is reduced and easier and more comfortable meanings can be imposed upon what doctors and nurses do to us (or *don't* do to us).

However, if we are seen to have only lost 'pregnancy tissue' or to have had only a 'heavy period', then the quality of the care we receive – both short-term immediate medical support and longer-term consideration – will be inadequate. Not *one* of us could relate to the description of miscarriage as 'slight cramping'. Indeed, as Chris Pope remarks in her article, 'The pain of a fruitless labour seemed much greater than the birth of my son 15 months later'.[6] Sentiments shared by many of us. These are difficult personal truths but, I would argue, infinitely more helpful in their honesty than the bland deceptions which pass for knowledge in this area. Ann described it in the following way:

> Each time I was told that as I was only two months pregnant, a miscarriage would be just like a heavy period with the same kind of slight stomach cramps . . . Then, early on Tuesday morning I

was awakened by severe pains in my stomach and back. I cried and cried as, over the next two hours, a pattern of contractions built up. The pain was intense and *nothing like a period.* [Emphasis added.]

The point about mentioning the inappropriateness of the language is *not* to intimidate other women, but to help us prepare more realistically for the demands which the experience might make on us. This is part of the same continuum within which women have claimed back areas of power, choice and responsibility in childbirth on the basis of revaluing what we know and demanding access to professional knowledge.

Therefore, it seems useful to conceptualise our expectations for sensitive prebirth loss care within these same terms. Suggesting this is not the same thing as compelling women to want this shared care in identical forms or indeed to want it at all! Many women we have spoken to talked for example of wanting 'to be looked after', 'to be in safe hands', of wanting to hand themselves over to 'the experts'. And this is an equally understandable desire which in the context of flexible and women-centred obstetric care should be available as a matter of course, giving women a sense of confidence that their differing needs for both competent and compassionate treatment will be met.

Finally, before leaving this section on language I want to suggest that it is not only the problem of medical terminology which acts to control the meanings around miscarriage and ectopic pregnancy. Equally unhelpful and often even more discomforting can be the common-sense language of our peers. This is partly because we have higher expectations of their understanding, only to be frequently disappointed by their apparent failure to embrace our experiences. Their distancing from us registered in the language of euphemism – 'your little trouble' (Janet) – is a safeguard to protect their own inadequacy and/or fear in the face of the death taboo. Thus all of us learnt very early on the coded message that we were meant to go away quietly and not to fuss.

But if medicine and common sense have converged in this way to resist our experience, then the sheer necessity of attending to our grieving business has compelled us to re-name miscarriage and ectopic pregnancy, pregnancy tissue, little bits of meat, products of conception, spontaneous abortion and so on, and instead insist upon their being named our 'lost babies'. I will show what a vital role this change played in opening up within us the permission to grieve, better able as a consequence to get a sense of self-knowledge and self-acceptance about these birth losses. I want to begin the next part, however, by discussing some of the reasons why it was that this business of failure weighed so heavily upon us. By understanding this and the equally powerful sense of guilt to which it seemed to be symbiotically attached, I think we can begin to uncover more of the paradoxical nature of prebirth loss and its compelling impact upon our sense of femininity.

The Sense of Failure: Feeling Fragile

One of the many ironies we had to face in confronting the facts of pregnancy loss was the acknowledgement that we felt vulnerable, lost, afraid, irrational, emotional and ill – in short, definitely fragile! Feeling this mix of emotions is one thing and owning up to it something else.

Many of us had after all, spent years working *against* this stereotype of the feminine. It was, and is, undermining of that hard-won self-confidence to find yourself complicit with, rather than critical of, this model of femininity.

In this situation we felt doubly exposed to the feelings of powerlessness, especially since we had been successful in other aspects of our lives. As Janet's and Sheila's accounts show in particular, the sense of autonomy and competence over the professional and personal aspects of your life are easily disrupted and challenged by the inadequacies you experience in coping with this private failure.

Janet, for example, felt herself hemmed in by the difficulties of wanting to be given support but singularly ill-equipped to ask for it, learning early on in her life that such supplication could be used to make her out as 'weak':

> Before the miscarriage I had learned that certain forms of expression at certain times were not helpful to me since they implied some victory over me – that I *did* have feminine weaknesses. The female stereotype put paid to most emotional expression in me.

Marilyn, too, similarly isolated in her hidden loss, could not ask for recognition and acceptance of her situation, because she had decided not to tell her work colleagues that she was pregnant.

She elected secrecy because she didn't want to open herself to criticism as a less than efficient worker. When she miscarried her third baby it was well and truly hidden. Here is how she describes the bind she was in:

> I still had my work. I enjoyed it. A freelance world – it was a place for survivors. I wore my smile like a mask. No one at work had known I was pregnant. There was no reason to know how I ached with emptiness (it was the other side of the coin) – I had always kept quiet for as long as I could when I was pregnant in order to be treated as a viable work unit for as long as possible.

Another of the difficult things to understand is the manner in which this private affair is somehow intimately connected with a fear that because we have not become mothers, we are incomplete in our femininity. And I think that one of the mechanisms which makes us afraid is precisely our own prior complicity in denying aspects of our femininity so that we are taken seriously in a male world as 'viable work units', in Marilyn's telling phrase.

I want to expand on this because for me it returns us to the heart of the paradox of pregnancy loss. Women have masses of evidence about the ways in which femininity is subordinated to masculinity. This power relationship is expressed in a variety of complex ways, ranging from ideologies which stress female passivity and male activity, through to practices which take their shape from these ideas, such as male sexual harassment and sexual violence. Central to female oppression is the core notion of the availability of female sexuality as the reward for men. Girls' and women's bodies are thus surveyed and controlled by the orthodoxies of media imagery; common-sense prescriptions about 'nice girls' and family and community notions of gender-appropriate behaviour and values sustain and encourage female passivity. It is important to recognise that these mechanisms work with and through race, class and age differentiations too.

Women who go against these formidable forces take risks with their self-esteem. Electing to express their femininity so that it encompasses the world of paid work puts them in a contradictory relationship to the stereotype of femininity as dependent, domestic and invisible (in the private space called home and family). If the world of public success is defined in antithesis to femininity, as I am claiming, then failure in the private sphere, for those women who have achieved public credibility, is very corrosive.

And it is only because femininity in this culture *is* principally defined as weakness that our struggles to be strong are taken as signs of masculinity. If we then revert to 'type' by becoming pregnant but lose the baby before term, we often experience ourselves as doubly devalued thereby. We are not 'proper' women. We have broken too many rules. These inner voices take their force from our always having to justify ourselves, to defend our right to be taken seriously, to function, in other words, in a male-centred world.

The psychological price to be paid for always feeling on the defensive is that you are particularly vulnerable to guilt. Here is how Sheila epitomises the complex feelings common to many of us about our experience:

> The possibility of problems had never before occurred to me. I knew things could go wrong in pregnancy but I felt I was one of the lucky ones who would sail through it with very little alteration from the norm (apart from getting bigger!). I was totally shattered. I was someone whose life revolved around bodily activity. I had worked hard to gain control in body action, to be aware of how my body moved and reacted to stimuli. I was fit and healthy. Now I felt I had lost all control of my body. I kept bleeding and there was nothing I could do about it . . . 'Pregnancy is not an illness'; you should be able to continue as before with slight limitations. I, who enjoyed fitness and activity, was now faced with terrible guilt. Had I brought on this miscarriage myself?

She then goes on to list her catalogue of 'selfish' actions – going on the tiring mountain expedition, overstraining herself, ect. – in short, to blame herself. If we have managed to struggle to achieve success in terms of our personal and working lives, we find ourselves particularly ill-prepared for this sort of failure, especially if we have always wanted to appear invulnerable and ready to challenge any negative assumptions about our capabilities – the 'superwoman' syndrome. We will have got nothing from the rosy pregnancy literature either, where 'failure' is confined to a sub-section on 'complications', if it is mentioned at all.

We seek reasons for feeling bereft. This imperative is determined by our desire to find an answer in the hope of restoring our bodies. If we can find something to blame, even if it is ourselves, then the puzzle is solved. It is this search for certainty which triggers our defensive guiltiness. Janet:

> And remembering that our close friend the doctor had once suggested that I was not in any physical state to have babies because I did not eat enough. My fault. And my father saying that I should not have lifted that sewing machine. My fault. And the obstetrician saying that nothing I did or didn't do would have caused this. Not my fault. But even so, it was my body that produced it.

A Sense of Guilt

This guilt battens on to all those areas in our life that we had previously sought to struggle for and it stems from the same source – our relative powerlessness in the face of all those social forces which resist our struggle for autonomy: the right to decent paid work – 'if only I hadn't done that extra . . .'; the right to reproductive choices – 'if only I had had *that* child'; the right to an active sexuality – 'if only I hadn't had sex'.

This sense of self-blame and consequent guilt is hardly news to us as women in this culture. We are already held responsible for our rapes, our children's delinquency, our husbands' drinking, our own murders even! And many people are happy to collude with our self-blame for prebirth loss too. A woman friend was telling her GP about her recent miscarriage only to be scolded: 'What a naughty girl, what had you done?'

Doctors, too, may seek to project their own incomprehension or inadequacy in the face of a miscarriage or ectopic pregnancy on to the woman by 'blaming the victim', especially if they feel that she is about to query whether their internal examination was a contributing factor.

An even more problematic instance is where a woman who has earlier exercised her choice over reproduction by having an abortion discovers that the instruments used to stretch the neck of the womb are now considered too clumsy or large, and may have contributed to a condition known as an incompetent cervix, which is thought to have caused the miscarriage. The sense of guilt that this diagnosis induces is more difficult to deal with, since a feeling of responsibility is inescapable.

This tendency for female self-blame was a constant theme in all of our spoken and written narratives about pregnancy loss – so much so that it almost seems to have the force of a biological imperative! One other way of placing it is by reference to a sense of particular isolation we feel as women in a society in which our values, concerns and experiences take second place.

Nowhere is this more true than in contexts where actual biological difference is central to the power play. In gynaecology and obstetrics, for example, where men ought to have the humility to recognise that difference at the very least requires them to learn from us what it feels like to possess or to lose a womb or a baby, we often find the exact opposite: an arrogant assertion of expertise which seems designed to pathologise the notion of difference altogether.

Despising our inside knowledge is part of a predisposition to view the female body as inherently suspect. You only have to recall the way menstruation is seen in this culture as the 'curse' to show something of the force of the taboo which surrounds our inner workings, while active female sexuality is a frightening thought.

Holding on to a sense of oneself as okay despite all this, calls for considerable resources, and while some of us might have managed to get by, and even to enjoy our bodies, our sexuality and sex, we experienced these hard-won gains as particularly vulnerable to being undermined. So instead of having bodily confidence, we are suspicious. At its strongest this can take the form of self-disgust, or in more benign terms, self-doubt.

We can thus suffer loss of confidence in our competence, our sexuality and our capacity to cope. Our minds may be full of fears about our future ability to 'get back to normal' or to conceive a child and carry one to term. After all, we have almost proved the case that women's bodies *are* suspect, and to add insult to feminist injury we find our feelings not only betraying us on this front but also containing the even more 'impure' thought that, for some of us, a loss of femininity itself is implicated in our loss of our child.

How are we to understand our condition if we have spent most of our adult lives contesting the practical equivalence of adult femininity with maternity, and yet when thwarted in *our* maternity we feel overwhelmed by irrationality, dependency and all those myriad emotions used against us in the past! Having been determined not to conform to the fragile norm of femininity and not to sacrifice our autonomy, we are inevitably shaken to find our consciousness of ourselves as women rendered full of unspeakable contradictions precisely about this involuntary lack of autonomy which these 'hidden losses' have revealed.

These feelings of guilt and so on can germinate not only because of the ignorance and mystification which passes for knowledge in birth and birth loss but also because there exists no alternative to this framework even within those feminist and radical cultures to which most of this book's contributors belong.

I think that our confusion in thinking through the impact of these losses was compounded by the disappointment of our expectation that the pro-women politics of the women's movement would have something useful to say about pregnancy loss. Although there is a tenacious resistance to the attempts to rescind the hard-won concessions on abortion, the inevitably reactive struggles to defend these gains have often led to the worst form of reductionism, in which complex issues are erased by the careless simplicities of poor politics and bad slogans.

Eileen Fairweather, in an insightful account of the difficulties facing reproductive rights campaigners, reminds us that in terms of first principles the campaigns are pro-choice, *not* pro-abortion. She argues persuasively that political sloppiness has often resulted in that important distinction being overlooked. She asks, 'Why do we make support for a woman's right to choose dependent on seeing the foetus as no more than a bunch of splitting cells? . . . the only way abortion will cease to be each woman's guilty secret is through our saying, without apology, "Yes, if necessary we put women first".'[7]

One of the main reasons why this book has been written is to address this simplification, to move the debate on to new ground, away from what seems to us to be an unhelpful tendency for the pro-choice politics (which we all explictly support) to converge with the medical discourse that makes statements about the status of the unborn child which fail to acknowledge its humanity. It is precisely because of this omission that the rhetoric of the 'right to lifers' makes such a powerful appeal, containing as it does this irreducible recognition.

Our feelings presented such a challenge to both the anti-feminist orthodoxy (that would have us split from our feelings and from women for whom abortion is their choice) and the cruder feminist-influenced mechanistic account of abortion (it's simply a matter of a D and C) that we were compelled to think again about our experiences and our choices in new forms which we debated collectively in the process of writing this book.

Hidden Loss first appeared in a climate in which women's access to safe, consensual treatment in the context of childbirth and prebirth loss had not been secured. Since then these issues have become even more politicised. In Britain moral campaigns singling out the so-called feckless single mother have attempted to police the family and acceptable forms of maternity, whilst in the US the Moral Right has literally armed itself against both those women who wish to have abortions and their supporters who continue to provide the services. The case for eternal vigilance about hard-won gains in women's health access and choice has never been more urgent.

Turning from the political context surrounding our maternity loss I would like to re-focus on the particularities of our guilt: I want to suggest that whilst guilt is a product of the general social conditions of women, it is also lived within the immediate contexts of our personal relationships. This may mean that events surrounding the conception of the child will be re-interpreted and questioned if that child is subsequently lost. Most of us found that a miscarriage or ectopic pregnancy necessitated a re-examination of our relationships, especially and crucially with our partners. We were forced to confront difficulties within the relationship, the acknowledgement of which might also be a further source of guilt: 'If only we'd been really together . . .' This is how I expressed it:

> Initially I felt essentially ambivalent. These two words do not do the least justice to the complex situation surrounding the conception. Looking back from a distance it seems that the imagined unadulterated joy was the absence at the heart of the memory.

If the baby is lost, this feeling of ambiguity can be readily used by the woman as having caused the loss. This leads not only to more guilt for failing in a relationship, but also to seeing the miscarriage as a punishment for ambivalent feelings, resulting in self-recrimination. One possible consequence can be to become convinced that 'it happened because I didn't really want the baby anyway', which can be self-destructive and punishing. Some psychoanalytic accounts of miscarriage seem to view it as the result of a woman's rejection of her pregnancy. And whilst I do not want to discount totally this thesis, it is important to register unease with a form of explanation which returns the problem to women, and to the most inaccessible part of them: the unconscious. It is important to remind the reader that medicine has been singularly unsuccessful in understanding prebirth loss, which makes it important to be critical of the all-too-easy loop that lays the blame on our own 'suspected' and 'suspect' bodies or minds.

Since the book first appeared in 1989, there has been other writing on the subject which has explored the emotional, social and medical–political contexts to prebirth loss[8] – these contributions have been written specifically to improve current practice amongst practitioners. And there have been important successes and developments in maternity care: Wendy Savage won her case against being sued for malpractice when she insisted on responding to her patients' needs; the Active Birth Centre flourishes; there is a general opening out of discussion to embrace alternative forms of delivery; from Odent's Water birth practices to the use of hypnotherapy and so on. In short a rather different climate now prevails – one that hopefully is more attuned to the rights of women to have informed choices about childbirth and care. We think in our own small way this book has contributed to the shift towards more women-friendly and flexible approaches.

I now want to draw all of the previous arguments together through a discussion of the right to grief and grieving.

The Right to Grief and Grieving

I feel that the best way to make sense of our stories is through the process of grieving, of acknowledging the 'emotional wreckage', to use Janet's phrase, as the essential starting point and basis for our recovery.

In one important way, though, we have to recognise that we don't actually get over the loss, not because we are preoccupied with morbidity, but because the experience has become part of our new selves. As Mary Anne said in a letter to me, 'We do not "get over" the loss; it is not to be thought of as an obstacle we jump but rather as part of us, and how do we "get over" being ourselves?'

Janet's account emphasises the transformative impact of this 'different sort of a death':

My miscarriage happened ten months ago. My body returned to its normal cycle of fertility quite soon. But my life, my relationships, my feelings, my emotions, my thoughts, my perceptions have not returned to my pre-pregnancy normality.

They never will. I am a different person, one I sometimes don't recognise. For me the loss of my baby was a loss of innocence. And that is a quality which cannot be regained.

Here Janet expresses our shared awareness that this brush with death fundamentally dislodges the complacency which used to pass for our view about existence. This loss of innocence reminds us of our own humanity and is eventually a source of a new form of self-knowledge, even if it costs us some pain in the process. Moving from the immediate crisis of coping with bereavement (which is redoubled in the emergency life or death situation of an ectopic pregnancy) to acceptance and to a position where you can contemplate another pregnancy takes time. We all felt we had to fight for time in the face of agencies and people who seemed to urge us on impatiently.

Part of the mismatch between their speedy insistence that we try again and our reluctance is the result of the profound failure of others to interpret our experiences in our language. And I mean this literally as well as metaphorically. If all we have lost is 'pregnancy tissue' or 'little bits of meat', then we *can* be seen as self-indulgent if we are wilfully holding back from another pregnancy.

Women are often unused to getting support: characteristically we are supposed to provide it. Asking for it for ourselves, for *as long as necessary*, seems daunting, especially if we are discouraged in the business by simple-minded injunctions to 'pull yourself together' (i.e. stop wanting support – be a woman and provide it); 'try for another as soon as you can' (another version of the same thing: stop brooding – start breeding); 'take better care of yourself' (i.e. it was all your own fault anyway, you shouldn't have a paid job, have gone out, and so on).

Searching for 'permission to grieve' is in itself very fraught and it can be further complicated by our sensitivity to people's ability to score points over this vulnerability. By being thought 'typically female', we have seen others discount our claims to be taken seriously, so we are ourselves sometimes reluctant to risk demanding what we need. Lesley, however, sees this demand for our grief to be recognised and shared as an authentic element in our progress through to a maturer sense of ourselves as women: 'I feel that cosseting ourselves, allowing our bodies and souls to heal in their own time, is not the same as succumbing to the stereotype of the congenitally feeble feminine woman.'

The important point in this is to do with time and the need for space to learn from the experience for *as long as it takes*. There is not set time when we are supposed to have recovered, although friends, lovers, colleagues and family may act as if there is. One of the most liberating things that the midwife who cared for me during my miscarriage said to me was, 'You will never forget this experience.' Looking now at these words they seem harsh, even punitive, and certainly I didn't fully grasp their significance at the time. But I now know that she was right, in the sense of recognising the importance and power which the event would hold for me.

These words gave me permission to admit the powerful cocktail of emotions which followed on from the event, immediately after the shock and numbness wore off. And you need the words to validate the experiences, otherwise you are reliant upon your own very depleted resources to do this – resources already fully committed to the business of getting by.

Picking up the Pieces

In the course of this chapter I have been concerned to understand the difficulties we had to face. I have tried to indicate the nature of the institutions (the family and hospital, for example) which operate with male-centred assumptions about women's roles, women's bodies and hence women's needs. I have shown how such assumptions work to repress our inside stories, which nevertheless have refused to go away quietly. Like women over the centuries we have each other as the first and the last resort. This analysis has sought to translate our private thoughts and feelings into a public language which demonstrates at a collective level our claim for serious attention.

I want to close by summarising how the paradox of the experience of prebirth loss is sustained. We go through the unalterable truth of it as a physical, internal and emotional experience, but it is also (and alterably!) determined by the inappropriate medical language, the insensitivities of 'common sense', and the damaging and self-limiting stereotypes of femininity as weakness and emotionality. We struggle against these to accept our own emotional state: to not dismiss it as self-indulgence, but to recognise it as the necessary first piece of evidence, an experience to which we must attend.

The principal point of this attention is to protect ourselves from the tendency to self-blame, guilt and the individual isolation which is both the consequence of self-destructiveness and part of its cause. It is by making our losses less hidden that we can begin to make our own language and to tell our own stories which we can then share with others. This book is part of that continuing process.

Part Four:
Coming Through and Going On

Introduction

Lesley Saunders

And now what? How is this experience, and the knowledge it brings, to be integrated into an individual's life? So far, this book has looked at what happened to women as they experienced the loss of their babies. Their pain, their anger at themselves and others, especially their doctors, have come through loud and clear. Their confusion and uncertainty, their grief, their efforts to understand this unexpected interruption to the pattern of their lives have surfaced in sorrowful and inspiring ways.

But we couldn't leave it there. It isn't enough to tell what happened, why it may have happened, nor even to contribute a feminist analysis of the event and its surround. In these concluding chapters we have brought together some practical suggestions for ways forward, ways of coming to terms with miscarriage and ectopic pregnancy that hold good irrespective of the inadequacies of relationships, the medical and health-care systems or social structures. Allusions are made, however, to the nature of those inadequacies and to how they might be addressed.

Marilyn notes the impact of miscarriage and ectopic pregnancy on women's lives generally, not just on their reproductive expectations. She goes on to consider how women may respond to both the idea and the fact of future pregnancies. Mary Anne takes the reader carefully through the processes and meanings of mourning. She shows how loss may acquire creative and constructive significance. I outline some therapeutic techniques and exercises of particular relevance to women in self-help groups.

Each of these chapters nods in the direction of the topic of women's mutual friendship and support in times of trouble. Far-reaching networks of acquaintance, colleague and intimate tighten and unwind as their needs bring women together or let them go their separate ways. A delightful instance of this occurred shortly before the book went to press for the first time. A woman called Helen Gould wrote to us from Australia: she told us about her experiences as a *doolah* or birth attendant in another aspect of her work – supporting women who were miscarrying. She recounted in detail how miscarriage may be an enriching and informative event. It enabled one woman, for instance, to resolve long-standing ambiguities in her primary relationships; another 'experienced a beautiful birthing at twelve weeks' pregnant'.

The implication of Helen's account is clear: as in birthing a live baby, so in miscarrying, the quality and meaning of the woman's experience can be profoundly influenced by the attitude of her attendants. Both these women felt their bodies could deal with what was happening with minimal medical intervention and found support for this belief. (They were in the early stages of pregnancy – late miscarriages and ectopic pregnancy are, of course, a different matter.) One woman was accompanied by her daughter throughout; she reports that the event had deepened and clarified their relationship. The other woman says:

> Having experienced a traumatic stillbirth in a hospital four years ago, where my baby was whisked from my sight, it was an event of great personal significance to actually touch, feel and see my unformed baby amongst the clotted blood. And then to be fortunate enough to spend the following two days being and talking with the same women (who supported me at the time) helped me resolve any negative emotional effects . . . My memories of that time are very warm and positive.[1]

We felt in 1988 that the time was ripe for women to campaign for the right and resources to miscarry in a more positive way, just as they had for giving birth in a more women-friendly environment. What, if any, signs of improvement can be discerned since then? Well, for example, a special service was held on 1 October 1994 in Guildford Cathedral to remember children who had died before they were born: a marker perhaps of how attitudes towards miscarriage and prebirth death are changing. There are, after all, many meanings of loss. A death is a death, whether of a loved companion or of an unknown half-formed foetus; but the nuances of mourning and recovery should not be limited, however they may initially be shaped, by institutions either of bricks and mortar or of social norms.

But, from the perspective of 1995, it seems that we also need to beware of over-sentimentalising our experiences. As we know from our cousins' situation in the USA, the notion of 'death of the unborn' has been used in an intentionally sensationalist way by fundamentalist and fascist right-wing groups to justify systematic harassment and abuse of adults, particularly women about to undergo terminations of pregnancy. We must therefore be very much on our guard for occasions and contexts when even our own words can be turned against us. There are enemies more dangerous than incompetent doctors or unsympathetic bureaucrats to contend with.

Future Pregnancies:
From Anxiety to Awareness

Marilyn Duker

To say that women change as a result of experiencing the loss of a baby through miscarrying or suffering an ectopic pregnancy may sound like a banal generalisation; of course all human beings are affected by the events life throws at them. They are affected by their successes and their failures, by their capacity to meet demands and expectations and to fulfil hopes they have for themselves and others. Prebirth loss is such an event. It is also one which, for a range of reasons discussed earlier on in the book, women are likely to experience as failure.

The impetus for this book about 'hidden loss' came from the very deep sense of disappointment and confusion felt by just a few of us, but as time went on we found those feelings shared by many more. Revealing our loss led other women not only to admit that they too had miscarried or had an ectopic pregnancy, but to 'confess' the extent of the grief or anger they suffered at the time – for the most part in silence. We found that even many years after their loss many women want to talk in detail about their experience and the way it affected their thinking about future pregnancies. Even those who were more glad than sorry that they had miscarried – because they had not been willingly pregnant, or because they felt ambivalent about having a child – admitted that their attitude towards pregnancy and birth had changed as a result of the event.

Our experience has been that however healed we've been physically, however much information and preparation we've been able to obtain through general antenatal care, ultrasound scans, genetic counselling and so on, and however much support we've received from people who've been loving, tender and understanding, we have not been able to confront with an easy mind the idea of becoming pregnant again.

It took four and a half years for me to be able to contemplate being pregnant again. I knew I wanted a child but I didn't think I could face being pregnant. I have had a lot of operations in my life. The ectopic pregnancy led to another, and then yet another operation still, when menstruating subsequently caused me so much pain. My marriage broke up too. All of this made it hard for me to come to terms with the fact that I had lost my baby. Emotionally it took me a long time before I could let that first baby go, before I could see a new baby not just as a replacement but as being in its own right. I've only got one [fallopian] tube left. I'm still afraid that something might go wrong. But at least now I can contemplate being pregnant again with more hope and courage.

There are obviously physical reasons why someone who has had an ectopic pregnancy might feel particularly apprehensive about becoming pregnant again. The fear that there may be only one chance left is based on reality. But the prospect of becoming pregnant again can also be daunting for a woman who's miscarried 'without complications', if it confronts her with too many un-resolved feelings about the pregnancy that, against her ex-pectations, went wrong.

It's when I find I'm expected to contemplate another pregnancy with equanimity that I mind – because I can't. It will be terrifying, walking on ice. I shall never have a pregnancy that is exciting, that is an interesting, innocent experience. I shall never have my first child. The next, if there is a next, will be my second child.

Nor is a successful pregnancy prior to the miscarriage or ectopic pregnancy any guarantee that the thought of subsequent pregnancy will be any easier. There are different strains; the problem has different perspectives:

I knew I was going to have to steel myself over becoming pregnant again. I wanted to complete my family. That was a very strong feeling, but I was frightened of the effort it was going to take. Not just the physical effort of enduring the wear and tear on my body, which I had begun to notice, but the effort of coping with the fear of miscarrying again. It was all the effort I knew I was going to have to put into keeping that fear down.

In each case our personal circumstances and experiences, as well as the feelings we had about wanting a child, tended to affect the speed with which we rushed into another pregnancy or the length of time we stalled. The effect of miscarriage on our self-confidence was part of the equation. We found such differences in the experience of other women too:

> It's hard to describe the sense of devastation and loss I felt. Even though I knew I would get pregnant again, I was not comforted. This baby, my first child, was not to be. We had been primed for that baby – planned for it, wanted it, made a space in our lives for it and then suddenly it was no longer there. The life we had created was now scraped away. We had to start all over again.

And by contrast:

> We tried to get me pregnant almost immediately but my body physically wasn't up to it. Our hasty efforts only served to make me more depressed; each time we thought we'd done it again, only to have our hopes dashed when I got my period . . . We're now trying to relax more about my getting pregnant – I try to do all the right things. We try not to build up our hopes every month, but it's hard not to.

Just as prebirth loss can sharpen a woman's awareness of her feelings about herself and her body, so it can also reveal a conflict between her reproductive, nurturing role and her non-domestic role. This conflict may be acute between the failure of pregnancy and subsequent conception, when a woman may feel she belongs to neither world:

> I found it was over the next few months that my preoccupation shifted slightly from what had happened to what might happen in the future. I felt totally compromised. I desperately wanted to become pregnant. I was obsessed with working out times of ovulation, dates, etc. I felt pressurised to try again soon. We wanted two children close in age, and time seemed to move rapidly. I had never wanted to extend my childbirth, childrearing years, I had so many plans for my future and my career. Did this mean I was selfish? Guilty yet again? I felt unable to settle to anything because I hoped to become pregnant, yet I was extremely frightened about becoming pregnant. I felt real fear and worry at the thought of a repeat performance of the miscarriage. I found these contradictory feelings very difficult to cope with.

If a woman becomes pregnant again, the lack of 'safety' she may feel about it can be undermining. Previously she may have juggled her time, talents and other resources as she tried to ease the tension between the demands of being a nurturer and her need to be an autonomous person, perhaps with an independent career. Many women do this with a remarkable degree of success; but the balance is often more precarious than it seems, or than the woman herself can admit. Any pregnancy may exacerbate the potential for conflict between her roles; a pregnancy which follows a miscarriage or ectopic pregnancy may do so all the more. Her commitment to motherhood, on the one hand, has been thwarted and her confidence in that role at least temporarily shaken. On the other hand, both her physical vulnerability and her interest in motherhood, which were simultaneously manifested in divulging her miscarriage, may, in the eyes of some, throw doubt on her entitlement to be taken seriously as a work colleague or as an employee. The woman herself may feel that neither role fits her present state.

I was enormously relieved when the consultant said he was going to admit me to hospital – then and there. I was going to be in for at least two weeks. The worry, the burden of myself and my anxiety about the baby was being lifted from me. But work was a problem. I didn't want anyone to know I was pregnant, still less that I was having a 'difficult' pregnancy. That kind of thing undermines credibility.

When they become pregnant again women may adopt strategies to deal with feelings that surround the possibility of failure. They need to find ways of shielding themselves, perhaps paradoxically by anticipating the worst:

When I became pregnant again some months later I didn't want to let myself think about it in case I had another miscarriage. I refused to tell anyone that I was pregnant in case everything went wrong again. Every hour I would rush off to examine my clothes for signs of blood and I was alert to the slightest twinges of pain. This was in spite of the fact that my doctor was very supportive and encouraged me to ring up about the slightest anxiety. My pregnancy continued – and I continued to worry. After the first 16 weeks had passed I began to let myself hope that this time things would be all right but I could never accept that they would be. I searched medical text books for causes of miscarriage at later dates and each time I went to the antenatal clinic I grew furious with the handouts which devoted a small paragraph to miscarriage, called it an 'unlikely' event, when I felt this was far from the truth.

Generally it's the early weeks which are the most nerve-racking, though for some women the anxieties continue beyond this stage:

With my new pregnancy I was excited and pleased as on previous occasions, but this was very much toned down with feelings of apprehension and fear as to what might happen. Consequently I felt unable to tell anyone except my husband that I was pregnant until past 13 weeks. Then I began to believe that perhaps everything might be all right. Even so, throughout this pregnancy I felt very uneasy. I found it hard to relax. I was continually expecting something to happen. For the first time I had frequent thoughts about problems associated with the baby. Suppose the pregnancy did progress satisfactorily – I was still afraid that there would be problems with giving birth or that the baby might be deformed. I kept most of these misgivings to myself but they made my pregnancy and the birth more of an ordeal than an experience to enjoy.

But if a woman is allowed to voice her fear, to acknowledge in power, this can bring its release, however stormy:

When I became pregnant again I was really sensible about taking care of myself. I was very organised about things like talking to my health visitor and getting advice about which GP would give me the kind of support I wanted. I felt confident in my consultant too. The care she gave me was excellent – but I just didn't know how scared I was. It was arranged for me to have a scan. This was more information. It would let me know things were all right. It was only when that machine came looming over me that the sheer dread took hold. It was then that I faced the unbearable possibility that the baby inside me might be dead. Facing it like that I just broke up – went to pieces, sobbing uncontrollably.

It helps if medical practitioners also understand the emotions that are surfacing:

If it was going to be ectopic it would have happened between the sixth and the tenth week. I don't think I realised the strain I was under until I saw the nurse for the blood tests and voiced my fears to her. She seemed to understand so well, allowed my fear legitimacy. She recommended I should see the doctor earlier than planned and told me I wasn't silly to feel afraid. I burst into tears when I left her – let the fear come out. I had some terrifying dreams around that time. I was really living on a knife edge.

Professionals who can provide support and reassurance of a non-patronising kind for women who have had a previous failed pregnancy are much valued:

Once I'd talked to my GP on the phone and then seen her and knew definitely it wasn't ectopic I felt I could begin to relax. But even then I couldn't take it for granted. I really don't mind all the antenatal visits – I get a bit more reassurance every time and a bit more faith.

He just sat there on the hospital bed and held my hand while I cried. He knew this baby was important to me. He was very patient and caring; just accepted that I was frightened of miscarrying again. This in itself was such an enormous relief.

Two weeks later only, but I was 14 weeks pregnant – more than three months and into a new phase of pregnancy. The consultant came and saw me just before I left hospital. 'A case of fear', she explained to her retinue, but she glanced at me and smiled and the tone of her voice carried the message that this was acceptable and understandable, a condition that would respond to treatment. But what treatment had I had? Rest, respite from myself, a caring environment at a crucial point in my pregnancy – and I felt better, reassured, hopeful. I cannot pretend that I felt entirely safe. There was still fear there. There were still so many long weeks ahead – but I could feel myself holding tightly on to hope.

One woman who had previously been able to encounter both male and female doctors with equanimity found, after a series of miscarriages, that she was quite unable to face a male GP. For the first time in her life she wanted to be dealt with only by a woman doctor. Others may also find their attitude towards doctors changes; perhaps they have more definite ideas about how they want to be cared for.

Women often give each other encouragement, simply by their presence and their understanding:

> There are women I now know who would understand. Should anything go wrong I know they'd be with me. Their support gives me the feeling that things might just go right.

But anxiety can and does stay with many women right up to the moment when their next baby is born:

> When I was pregnant the second time, I felt sure I would miscarry again. For nine months I willed my muscles so efficiently to hold the baby in lest it drop out on the pavement (despite what I knew about the causes of miscarriage) that it took two days of hard labour to get him out!

Frequently they harbour worries that the miscarriage they suffered might have been caused by some abnormality of the foetus and they fear that the new child may be born handicapped.

> The first thing I wanted to know when Thomas was born was, 'Is he all right?'

Another woman described how her behaviour during labour itself was a release of previous feelings:

> I was in floods of tears and my husband had to explain that they were tears of relief at being in labour, not of pain. And it was true. The time was right for these contractions this time. I was able to relax, let go. Whatever the pain, I could take it all for this baby. The labour was quite long. The cervix took a long time to retract, which had never happened when my other children were born, but I didn't care, even when the contractions grew really excruciating. I wanted this baby alive. For that I would suffer anything. The fear was still with me right until the moment he was delivered.

Occasionally the experience of miscarriage can live on after the birth of a live and healthy baby; fears can sometimes be reawakened with subsequent pregnancies:

> It was really quite early on that panic began to eat me up. I was

quite alarmed that fear should still have this strong hold on me, even though I'd given birth since that last miscarriage. There'd been some doubt at the time whether that had been ectopic, though fortunately it hadn't. Now it was that particular fear which was overwhelming me. I was checked out and the foetus was in the right place, but I was still gripped with fear that this was really an ectopic pregnancy. In the weeks that followed I found myself having to concentrate tremendous energy into recalling that picture – the foetus growing exactly where it should be. I guess the trouble was that I couldn't take pregnancy for granted any more. Because I was scared, I ate and put on far more weight than I should have done. It wasn't until I felt her alive, separate, tiny naked body against mine that I felt safe.

There are many women who have suffered miscarriages or ectopic pregnancies and who, for a variety of reasons, never carry a healthy baby to term. Some of them may carry the sadness of that loss for the rest of their lives; opportunities to express grief, despair, rage or any other strong feeling about it may have occurred only rarely and in a limited context. A great deal more support for such women needs to be forthcoming.

As giving birth and entering into motherhood is a threshold in a woman's life, so too is the experience of pregnancy loss. It is a threshold where the crossing is hidden, but it may likewise make a profound difference to the way a woman lives her life in future. What kind of difference is for each woman to discover. One woman described it like this:

For me it seems that miscarriage is something that makes a difference to how one is. It was something that changed me, quite fundamentally. A part of me died. It was a brush that I had with death. I find I can no longer take life for granted. This was a very intense feeling in the early stages after miscarrying and it has subsided, but it is still there. Nor will pregnancy ever be the same experience again. I have lost my nonchalance there. Previously birth had been a simple notion. Now it holds the possibility of death. Before, I was able to take the way my body functioned for granted. Now I am horrifyingly aware that it will not always do what I want it to . . . Life has become even more precious than it was before. Over the two years that I kept miscarrying I think I grew old. And those two years also seem to be missing. There's a gap there – two years of my life when I don't seem to have been alive. Even now, four years later, I am still coming to terms with this: trying to understand how I came to be 36 so soon; trying to catch up on the living that I've missed.

Letting Go and Holding On

Mary Anne Speakman

It takes an awful long time to sort it all out, doesn't it? But if my experience is anything to go by, it's possible to get there in the end, or at least to continue to get there. Recovery is not a linear process, but each time you go down a bit, you go up a bit further the next time.

This extract from a letter written by a woman, three years after she had lost her baby, to another woman more recently bereaved, sums up the essence of this chapter. How can we make sense out of the confusion, uncertainty and grief experienced when we suffer a pregnancy loss? What can we do to ease the pain and resolve the conflicting emotions we feel?

We have called the process of understanding *letting go and holding on*. We mean by this gradually becoming able to let go emotionally of the baby who is no longer inside us physically, but to retain the memory as a positive part of our lives. The experience becomes integrated into our lives as we are able to move forward with new understanding. Physical and emotional recovery do not usually go hand-in-hand; the former commonly occurs more speedily than the latter. It is important to recognise that both types of recovery are linked, though, and also that recovery is a process. It is unlikely that there will come a specific moment when one will wake up and say 'Right, that's all over – I'm never going to think about that again.' It takes time to recover. No one can say how long it will take because it's different for everyone, and different feelings surface at different times. Feeling physically better will help, but it's extremely common to feel emotionally vulnerable months, even years, afterwards, and especially at significant times, such as the anniversary of the loss or when the baby's birthday should have been.

However, there will come a time when it is possible to look back on what happened with composure, with the bitterness and sadness lessened in intensity if not completely gone, having reached a stage when it is possible to let go of the baby and the depth of the experience of loss. Holding on is, paradoxically, part of the process of letting go. It means being able to integrate the experiences of loss and grief into life, to learn about oneself from them, even to gain something positive from the process of coming through what has been a stressful and painful phase in one's life. Thus, the experience is not lost for ever, shut up in an unconscious part of the mind, but can be turned into something more constructive, however unlikely this would appear at the time of loss.

Recovery does not equal forgetting, but it can mean personal change and this can be experienced positively:

> I do know what you mean about 'recovery' – I don't think one does really recover or 'get over it'. After all, what has happened to us has become a fundamental part of ourselves and we never 'recover' from being ourselves, do we? I think the pre-loss self and the post-loss self are both very much parts of the same self, but you can't go back to the other self, because the experience has been like a staging post on a journey at which we've been forced to stop and think and find out more about ourselves. Whilst I wouldn't have freely chosen to stop, or go through my loss, I sometimes do feel that it has forced me to confront more aspects of my self than I would otherwise have done, and so, too, to realise more fully what being a woman means to me. And this, in the end, is a positive and constructive thing, though it's taken a long time to see it like this.
>
> (Letter from Mary Anne to Valerie)

The Process of Grieving

Before we consider specific suggestions for ways of coping with pregnancy loss, it is worth looking at how the emotional effects of miscarriage and ectopic pregnancy may be experienced. Women often feel a lot of pressure to 'get over it' quickly, expressed in phrases such as 'pull yourself together', 'stop moping around' or 'don't get morbid'. Consequently they often do 'put a brave face on it', even when inside they feel their world has totally disintegrated. This is particularly so when the miscarriage was early and few people even knew they were pregnant. So there comes the added worry that what is being felt is somehow weird, an overreaction or self-indulgence. It's very important to be able to express feelings, to share them with others, and to understand that the range of emotions experienced is not silly or bizarre. Feeling sad, angry, bitter, being excessively tired, losing your appetite, not sleeping well are common responses shared by many women in this situation. The letters written by the women in our group often expressed this. For example,

> I don't know whether you are still physically recuperating, as well as emotionally shedding and healing. I'm sure it's very important to take ourselves seriously about this, and really not feel there's an obligatory time by which we should be 'better'. I feel that consulting ourselves, allowing our bodies and souls to heal in their own time, is not the same as succumbing to the stereotype of the congenitally feeble, feminine woman. After my miscarriage, I sensed that other people were telling me to get back to work, to stop brooding – maybe that's what worked for them, but I wanted to *know* what I felt, to experience it so that it wouldn't, at some future time, lay me low with unresolved anguish or anxiety. And because we have a *right* to grieve over what we lose and slowly incorporate what we've learnt.

(Letter from Lesley to Valerie)

Death is commonly hidden away in our society; people tend to stigmatise the bereaved as if their loss and suffering is catching and therefore often deny the depth of feeling and the length of time needed for full acceptance to occur. But mourning is a psychological necessity, not self-indulgence or weakness. There may be days a long time after you thought you'd got over the worst when you feel like crying all the time, you can't sleep or just feel low and unable to cope. However, it's worth remembering that each time you go downhill a bit, it's not so far as the last time.

Stages of Mourning

Losing a baby through miscarriage or ectopic pregnancy is a bereavement, so it is quite natural to feel grief. What we have lost is far more than just a baby, for that baby represents so many other facets of our lives, hopes and fears, and will be different for each of us. We have lost a much-wanted daughter or son, who might also have been a sister or brother and grandchild; we have lost proof of our ability to conceive, which may be especially hard to accept if we have experienced fertility problems; we have lost a belief in the reliability of our bodies; we have lost the outward evidence of the bonds between us and our partners; we have lost something which we may have felt ambivalent about; we have lost a physical part of ourselves.

Coming to terms with the bereavement will involve working through three main stages of mourning that are common to anyone experiencing loss, whether it be the loss of a loved one through death or separation, loss of a bodily organ or limb (the fallopian tube in the case of an ectopic pregnancy), or loss of a baby at whatever stage of pregnancy. These 'stages' are not, however, experienced as distinct entitites with clear beginnings and endings but merge into each other, with symptoms overlapping or re-emerging, and their length varies with each individual. It is probably only retrospectively that one can see there was a pattern to one's mourning, to the 'grief-work' that needs to be done to achieve acceptance. If you are somewhere in the middle of your grief-work now, the idea of stages may not make much sense, but it may help to realise that others feel the same, or react the same, as you recognise symptoms applicable to you.

Grief is perhaps most intrinsically marked in the early days by sudden and periodic pangs of grief, when the lost baby and all she or he represented is acutely missed. These usually reach a peak five to 14 days after the loss and then gradually decrease, appearing only when one is reminded specifically, by, for example, seeing a friend who is still pregnant, or walking past a shop selling baby clothes.

The first hours and days are characterised by shock and disbelief. Typical of this time is a sense of numbness, of living in a vacuum, and it is common to attempt to deny what has happened to protect oneself from the truth. So a woman who has miscarried may pretend for a while that she is still pregnant. Another reaction to the loss is a feeling of needing to search for the baby, as if it had simply been mislaid somewhere. One woman spoke of her hesitancy to leave the hospital. 'I recall feeling anxious on leaving the hospital: a tremendous feeling of "leaving something behind". I didn't want to go until I'd found it.' One aspect of the searching is a preoccupation with going over in one's mind the events leading up to the miscarriage or ectopic pregnancy. Part of the reason for this is to try to find the lost baby, and part is to see whether there wasn't anything else that might have been done; in other words, seeking reassurance that one was not to blame.

During the second phase, it is as if the numbness has worn off and the reality of what has happened has to be faced. Behaviour may be very odd at times, and you may feel you're going mad. You're not. Mood swings, surges of intense activity followed by periods of lassitude, becoming forgetful or more irritable than usual, going out for a walk or to the shops and then forgetting where you are going or what you needed to buy, feeling no longer capable of driving the car or catching a bus – all of these sorts of seemingly irrational ways of behaving are perfectly normal reactions to loss. This is a time of coming to accept that the miscarriage or ectopic pregnancy really did occur, that 'this baby will never be', that this pregnancy will not bear fruit, and that life will never be the same again. This requires an enormous amount of adjustment but this stage must be worked through if the loss is to be accepted.

Women sometimes speak of this time as if they were on a seesaw which goes up and down rather unpredictably:

> I can be chugging along quite buoyantly and purposively and some chance event can trigger off a set of memories and consequent pain, and before I realise it – I'm sobbing convulsively. (Valerie)

The mask which people usually wear to hide raw emotions is worn very thin by a painful miscarriage experience and women are less able to hide their feelings or ignore the messages of related events. It's a sad irony that before we miscarried, we never noticed how many baby shops, babies and pregnant women there were around.

> I still cry and am upset by anything that is associated with the death of children or with miscarriage. I am still emotionally volatile. I feel that others, however, expect me to have got over it all. Even a month after the final medical, physical event, I felt that my feelings of utter misery and sadness at the sight of so many pregnant women were unsociable. (Janet)

As well as feeling their bodies let them down by 'failing' to carry the pregnancy to term, women sometimes find their bodies take a long while to adjust to not being pregnant again. This, together with nerve endings that feel sensitive in the extreme, can be quite a lot to cope with in itself.

> I became very tired, in fact I was convinced I was anaemic and

went through a blood test to eliminate that as a source of my feebleness – interestingly enough, I began to feel a great deal more energetic after that, though not as bouncing as I like to remember myself. Also, I've been experiencing womb turnings and greatly increased menstrual loss and massive PMT [premenstrual tension] sensitivities . . .

There was a time when I could hardly bear to put myself in stressful situation – I shook, and felt my muscles tighten all over my body as if my cheekbones would perforate my skin with the tautness of the facial tension . . . I felt as if I was living life at such an intensity that my colour perception, too, was affected, as was my aural receptivity. It was like being 150 per cent alive in some souped-up state and, when I wasn't in a totally friendly environment, I thought that at times I would explode with the bottled up tension of coping with so many contradictions. Predominantly I kept thinking to myself, 'How can the world keep ticking over so dully when I am in such a state? Why don't people notice? How can we bear the pretences?' And I kept thinking of that beautiful passage in George Eliot's *Middlemarch*, when she speculates that if human beings were to listen to that sound of pain they 'would die of that roar that lies the other side of silence'.

(Letter from Valerie to Mary Anne)

This sense of isolation is one that many women we talked to mentioned. Janet, for instance, said, 'I knew that I was experiencing it all alone. I felt totally alone.' It seems impossible that life goes on as normal, when the woman who has just miscarried has been through one of the most difficult times of her life. It's hard for friends to realise the intensity of the experience, unless they've been through it themselves, especially if the pregnancy was in its early days and not widely known about. Even when the miscarriage occurs later, people find it hard to allow open mourning, are uncertain what to say or how to show sympathy and, sadly, often resort to saying or doing nothing. With ectopic pregnancy, the concern for physical recovery can effectively mask the grief felt for the lost baby and lost tube. However, even if the grief can't be fully shared, it is vital that other people try to *accept* that the woman is grieving and let her do so, in her own time. By accepting, they can confer validity on her experience and not discount it. It's far better to say, 'I'm sorry' than nothing at all. Janet went on to say:

> The physical experience is a woman's, so why should I expect the emotional experience to be shared fully or even understood properly? Why should I imagine that anyone would understand that I can grieve for so long over the death of a seven and a half week old foetus? In the end, I don't expect anyone who has not experienced it to understand. But I want them to *accept* that this is the case, that it is with me still and rampages from time to time. I need my experience to be accepted as valid. Not necessarily understood, but recognised as proper.

It is very important that this acceptance of the experience as valid is given, otherwise the process of mourning may be halted or slowed down. One woman, for example, who found she had little support or understanding at the time of her ectopic pregnancy, suppressed her grief at the time, only to find her unresolved feelings re-emerge later:

> First of all when my marriage broke up and then when I had to go into the hospital again, to the same ward where I had lost the baby, to have an operation on my ovary which, tubeless, didn't seem to be able to function on its own. That was really when I allowed myself to grieve and admit my sadness.

This is really a form of buffer strategy when only certain aspects of loss can be dealt with at one time. New issues may only be dealt with if sparked off by some external event. For example, Marilyn wrote,

> Another, quite different miscarriage and two children later, I thought that it would have healed. But even five years later I have wept uncontrollably as I scribbled this down, and unaccountably wept again into the typewriter as I made it legible.

This second stage of mourning may last for weeks, months or even years. It depends on the circumstances of each individual woman, the help and support she has received, the degree of acceptance for her grief, her physical recovery, the intensity of her longing for a child. Eventually, though, she will enter the final stage, at the end of which her mourning is completed, and she will have recovered from the pain of her loss.

This is a time of burial, when the woman lays to rest her images of her lost baby and the version of herself with which she began the grieving process. Maybe she will be helped by making a memorial for her baby or by sharing experiences in a self-help group. She accepts that the baby she miscarried is never going to be born and, whilst not forgetting that baby, is able to redirect her energies to other aspects of life and to integrate her experience into her life. The experience will have changed her, but it is possible to come through with something positive at the end.

I just want to reassure you that your feelings of uncertainty about who you are now, what sort of a person, etc., will gradually sort themselves out. You're discovering parts of yourself that you didn't know were there because the situation in which they would show hadn't occurred. But the other known parts are still there. It will take time to find out how the different aspects link together, but that *will* happen. I learnt to understand myself better and also to accept the parts of me that I don't actually like very much and I feel that has been a good thing . . . that positive outcome is really worth hanging on to.

(Letter from Mary Anne to Valerie)

It may seem impossible at the time that you'll ever reach this point, but there are ways of coping that will aid recovery and in the last part of this chapter I'll be looking at some of the strategies we came across whilst writing this book.

Partners, Children and Grandparents

The way in which those around us react to our pregnancy loss can do much to determine how quickly we start to heal. Some women find their miscarriage or ectopic pregnancy brings them closer to their partners, although their relationship may have been changed by the experience. Some feel their partners do not always share their perceptions or appreciate the significance of, for example, anniversaries. The fact that the physical experience is a woman's and that, maybe, the emotional impact cannot be shared fully with a male partner can be a source of resentment.

Some men acknowledge that they do not experience a sense of losing a baby as deeply as their partners. Sheila's husband wrote,

The loss hadn't really affected me. I was too tied into Sheila's physical condition and her feelings to think much about 'a baby' being 'lost'. The baby had no identity for me as such – it had not been in my body in that sense, so it was not 'there' – but Sheila was 'there' . . . My own personal feelings were dominated by a deep sense of my own inadequacy to help her.

However, although the loss may not be experienced in the same way, there will still be a grieving process to go through and the more that feelings can be shared between partners, the more support and help they can give each other.

When the woman already has children she (and her partner) will have to try to explain what has happened to them as well as cope with their own feelings. When the children were unaware that a baby was expected it may be a case of explaining the mother's absence through hospitalisation and giving reassurance of her return. When the children were aware of the baby they will also have to be told of her or his death. It is never easy to explain illness and death to children, for whom the event signifies the end of certainty in their world and may lead to fears for their own survival. It is generally thought best to explain what has happened as simply and honestly as possible whilst giving constant reassurance. Explanations can always be amplified later when the child is older. Allowing the child to see you are sad gives the child permission to grieve too, and shows that it is quite acceptable to show your emotions.

There are additional issues to handle when the pregnancy loss is in the context of a twin conception and one of the children survives. The emotional and social consequences of this rare but important circumstance have been recently sensitively explored in *Coronation Street*. The mixture of grief and joy; of a loss and a celebration coincident within one experience forces home the contradiction at the heart of the experience with particular and poignant power. Such feelings are likely to be evoked especially at birthdays and can complicate the way you might feel. It is quite understandable if there are ambiguities at these times – of feelings concerned wtih 'what might have been'.

The other people most likely to be closely affected are the parents of the woman who has lost the baby and of her partner. Like

Sheila's husband, they may not immediately perceive the loss as a baby, being bound up in their concern for the well-being of the woman. Experiencing it as the loss of their grandchild may not come about till later. One woman wrote,

> My mother had come to look after me when I came out of hospital. We talked about how I felt but not about her feelings, though I sensed her deep worry over me. Shortly after her return home she wrote to say that she had suddenly realised that it was not only my child that was lost but her first grandchild, and that she had sat down and wept. Sharing her feelings with me then was so important and brought us so much closer together.

It is important to think through whether you might want to talk about your lost child/children to any subsequent surviving children. There can be no prescriptions about this. However, it is the opinion of most of the contributors to this book that since miscarriage and ectopic pregnancy are nothing to be ashamed of and are not our 'fault' then telling one's children can be a way to raise with them feelings and views which you have about the past. Equally such sharing can sensitise them as well as inform them that prebirth loss is much more common than the sources of information about the experience suggest.

Strategies for Coping

People who have experienced bereavement often feel the need for withdrawal, a time to stay indoors more, to just *be* rather than always be *doing* something. Our culture gives little recognition of this need and it is particularly difficult for women to find space for themselves as they are expected to be available to service others' needs and to be able to cope. Most do, despite the odds stacked against them, but managing to carry on living something approaching an ordinary life whilst trying to come to terms with your feelings takes a lot of energy in itself. So the first thing is to look after yourself. If it is possible, pamper yourself by getting up late, going to bed early if you feel like it, having a rest in the afternoon if you can. If you've lost your appetite, just eat what you can, even if it's not much, for your appetite will come back eventually. If you find yourself taking refuge in the fridge and overeating, well, try not to overdo it, but don't try to cope with a rigid diet at the moment. If you have children, consider whether you could ask someone to care for them for the odd afternoon to give yourself the space you need. Cosset yourself a bit and don't feel you have to apologise for 'not being all there'.

As well as looking after yourself, there are several other things you may find helpful.

Talking it over

However much you are able to talk over your loss with your partner, family or friends, there may come a time when you feel the need to gain support from other women who have had similar experiences. You may come across them by chance – it's surprising how many women you discover have had miscarriages or who know of someone who has when you admit to it yourself to colleagues at work, to someone in the doctor's waiting room, even to the lady at the local corner shop.

You can also contact several organisations which may be able to put you in touch with other women in your area. The Miscarriage Association and the National Childbirth Trust are two such groups, or there may be a local women's centre or women's health group (see Appendix 5 for addresses). It's worth asking your GP, midwife or health visitor, too. You could even write a letter to your local paper or the newsletter of a national organisation you may belong to – that's how our group got together – and you can always use a box number to preserve confidentiality. Having found one, two or several other women who are willing to listen and help, you may find it sufficient to share your experiences, compare them and lean on each other for support. You may want to try something more structured, such as self-help therapy, and Lesley provides more information on this in the next chapter. But do remember that the other women will want you to listen to them, too. The exact balance of listening and talking will depend on the stage of mourning each individual has reached, but the success of your meeting will depend on the degree of reciprocity you can all achieve.

You may decide to keep your group small and to let it last just as long as you yourselves need it, but groups sometimes evolve into a longer-term commitment, with the original members providing a support network for women more recently bereaved. Help can be given by telephone or in drop-in sessions at a local centre or an individual's home. When this happens, it is really valuable to establish good relations with local hospitals, GPs and other health professionals, so that they will not feel their toes are being trodden on but will give their support and refer their patients to the group. It is worth applying to borough councils, borough lotteries and local industries for funds, and it may be possible to do a course on listening skills or helping the bereaved with a local National Childbirth Trust branch or bereavement group.

You may prefer to seek professional help. The obvious person to turn to first would be your GP who, if unable to help you directly, could refer you to a therapist or counsellor. You could seek help privately, especially if you wanted to see a feminist therapist. You could contact the Women's Therapy Centre.

Seeking help from alternative medicine

There are now many more opportunities to use alternative therapies within the context of mainstream provision. Even the change of name to 'complementary therapies' suggests a new accommodation between classic medicine and its 'rival'. In part this has been due to the recognition of the failure of Western medicine to treat certain chronic conditions – for example, back pain sufferers record much greater success rates with osteopathy than with general practitioner interventions. In a climate of cost-cutting and economic rationality, the government has not been slow to incorporate complementary therapies when it has felt the weight of the economic argument. Prince Charles' endorsement of homeo-pathy appears to have worked to legitimise the regimen and the general growth of interest in New Age ideas, eco-friendliness and 'healthy lifestyles' have all played their part in prompting, in often incoherent and uneven ways, a range of treatments. It should therefore prove much easier to access these now than in the late eighties. The general incorporation of alternative therapies into the mainstream has reduced costs for practitioners and brought their services within the range of people on moderate incomes. Some forms of complementary therapy can even be obtained on the NHS. Many large London hospitals are providing a variety of treatments and pregnancy preparation classes in response to the changing culture of customer responsiveness, but these may be less available in rural and under-populated parts of the country. A couple of women in our group had experienced homeopathy and osteopathy and had found these therapies enormously beneficial, which is why we decided to include a mention of them here. Other relevant therapies are acupuncture and herbal medicine. The initial reason for visiting alternative medical practitioners was physical – a bad back, knee, painful periods, a general feeling of being unwell – but it was found that these therapies not only eased these physical symptoms but also released emotional energy as well, greatly helping the healing process. Alternative medicine recognises there is a close relationship between the body, the mind and the spirit. A problem in one affects the others, and healing, too, will occur at all levels.

An alternative practitioner can play a supportive role to traditional medicine in the case of an emergency. For example, a homeopath can give remedies to speed the healing process after the shock of surgery or to aid wound repair. However, the chronic situation is where treatment is more usually applicable. A common occurrence is when a woman seeks the help of alternative medicine months or even years after her pregnancy loss. Long after the emotions of grief have been experienced, the body can still bear witness to them in its residue of tight muscles or organic disturbances. A traumatic event can leave its mark on the body structure and function. For example, there might be adhesions developing from scarring round the site of the fallopian tube (removed as a result of an ectopic pregnancy), which can lead to painful periods or pain during sex. As well as easing such physical symptoms, the alternative medical practitioner can help the woman to relate these to her feelings, and give guidelines on diet, exercise and coping with stress factors in the environment.

Even if you do not wish, or are unable, to visit a practitioner, there are other ways of exploring the relationship between mind, body and soul and therapy can help the healing process, for example by examining your dreams. Emotional pain causes tension which is reflected in your dreams. One woman found that most of her dreams contained journeys, which she realised was not strange at all, because she saw her process of recovery from the time of her loss as a journey through the new and alien territory of painful emotions and fears.

Creating rituals

In comparison with other cultures and other times, our society has largely done away with the rituals associated with death and bereavement. People who have lost a relative or friend say that the lack of ritual makes grieving harder. There is a need for a funeral service, for memorials, for black bands on the arm, for notices in the newspaper. These outward signs help the long-term acceptance of death and adjustment to living without the loved one.

There is no ritual at all when the loss is caused by miscarriage. There is no death certificate, rarely a burial service, rarely even a visual picture of the baby to remember. People may not even know there has been a death. We have found it can help to create your own rituals. Writing the baby a story or a poem could be one, for that approximates a kind of obituary. One woman made a scrapbook in which she wrote down what had happened and included a photograph of herself taken around the time of the miscarriage, her hospital wristband, and the cards and letters which people had sent. It may be important to create a burial for the baby. Here, one woman describes her experience:

I've had this awful image of the baby struggling, trapped in the tube, and then instead of achieving freedom in the warmth of the womb, being out alone and cold on a clinical chrome table, and then into an incinerator. My friend asked me where I would like to see the baby, and I described a field of corn and poppies with trees and blue sky and sun. A very warm picture, and the symbols of fertility, instead of death. Burial instead of cremation which I am very against, personally. She suggested that I draw these pictures, to symbolically give the baby a resting place.

I went out and bought some pastels and drew three pictures, one of the baby on the table, one of the cornfield with the baby lying there, and one with the grass grown over. It was a very painful experience; I haven't cried so much for a very long time but now I feel an overwhelming sense of relief and lightness, and the beginnings of a resolution. I can now bring to my mind the cornfield and the image is becoming stronger all the time. I am thinking now of embroidering a tapestry of the cornfield which will be a long-term project and a kind of memorial. Also, I want to get a yellow rose bush for the garden so I can see it from my study.

Pruning the rose bush became a gentle way of keeping in touch, particularly at the time of anniversaries. It's not uncommon to think, 'she or he would have been five, six, seven years old now', and this kind of memorial can be a useful way of reflecting on sad memories. As it turned out, the rose bush was the kind where the flower bud stayed tightly closed for some time, before blossoming out all at once and then as swiftly shedding its petals, which seemed a very appropriate, though inadvertently chosen, type of rose to have planted.

Sometimes there is a need to give life to something before you can accept death, and the symbolic rituals of creating a tapestry, making a collage, writing a poem or planting a rose bush can be the way of 'breathing life' into the baby in order to bury her or the pain of her loss.

The Right to Mourn

Finally, you may need to be assertive in establishing your right to be sad, to grieve, and to adopt any of the strategies we have suggested above. You do have a right to mourn and to have this need respected by other people. You have the right to ask that other people respond to your needs and the right to express your feelings in ways that will not violate the dignity of others. (At some point, you might find it helpful to read a book on assertiveness training or attend a course; see Appendices 2 and 5.)

It is particularly hard for women to assert their need to grieve without being accused of being weak, sentimental, over-emotional, selfish. We learn from our earliest days that we are more likely to be liked (and, therefore, accepted) if we are happy, if we laugh and smile and keep our anger, frustrations or sadness hidden away. Janet expresses the impact of these messages on the expression of our loss very clearly:

> If I collapsed in tears or depressive passivity, I felt that it would be misinterpreted as unnecessary wallowing, as game-playing, as sympathy-seeking . . . Emotional expression is a difficult issue. Before the miscarriage, I had learned that certain forms of expression, at certain times, were not helpful to me, since they only elicited responses which seemed to imply some victory over me, that I *did* have 'feminine' weaknesses. The female stereotype put paid to most emotional expression in me . . . Not wanting to be treated as feminine meant not displaying behaviours which elicit such treatment. Tears are such behaviour. Voluble anger is another. But the experience of miscarriage has an emotional

impact which cannot be repressed so easily. And so I had to learn that if I were to cry or to be depressed or sad or have extreme responses to apparently insignificant events, then I would also have to explain myself, interpret myself against female stereotypes. To express my feelings was to take on a battle.

It is one of the inconsistencies of being a woman in our society that we are expected to cope, to smile and laugh, to be in control, whilst the outward expressions of not coping, of sadness and grief are denigrated as feminine weakness. It makes our loss an even greater tragedy when we have to fight for the right to mourn, as sadly, many women do. We need our experience to be recognised as valid, even if it is not necessarily understood, and so we should not have to hold back from expressing our need to grieve, even if it means repeating that over and over again. Being assured of the validity of our experience by those close to us, and accepting it ourselves, is perhaps the most important part of the grieving process, of being able to let go of the pain whilst integrating our loss into the rest of our lives.

Acknowledgment

I would like to thank Catherine Henderson, a homeopath and osteopath, for her help and advice in the writing of the section on seeking help from alternative medicine.

Dreams and Dramas:
Self-Help for Prebirth Loss

Lesley Saunders

The exercises in this chapter contain ideas for exploring issues and feelings, using a variety of well-tried techniques from women's self-help therapy. They are not holy instructions or tests that you pass or fail, merely suggestions to utilise where they seem to fit. There is, of course, a far wider and deeper range of therapeutic approaches than I have outlined. Some women may want to seek help on individual basis; some relevant addresses are given in Appendix 5.

What I Feel is Real

To lose a baby before she is born is to experience something which is both peculiarly private and common to countless other women. The tendency for each woman to have to contain the experience within herself means that, although a chance remark between friends may lead to conversation and mutual sympathy, the sharing of deep pain and anger is rarely reached. The resources for healing are there, but untapped.

Other chapters in this book explore the potential for prebirth loss to induce a sense of failure – our bodies did not behave in the way they were meant to. Part of dealing with that may be to reappraise the roles that society and biology between them seem to have imposed on women. A woman who has become pregnant is put directly in touch with her society's ideas and images of womanhood; losing the pregnancy opens a gulf between these stereotypes and her individuality. It is a disturbing and painful opportunity to own more of herself.

This is a step which not every woman will need or wish to take. For those who do, there are ways to assist the process. Perhaps the very first move is – to stay still. To hang on to one's actual feelings and subjective understanding, however contrary these may be to what is expected. We can actively seek images for these feelings and sensations if the conventional ones don't fit. It may be difficult, for example, to make a connection between diagrams of a uterus or foetus and one's experience of sexuality, pain, loss.

Describe in writing what happened. Miss nothing out. Don't concern yourself with style or punctuation. Recreate for yourself this event and what it meant. Go on until you've finished.

Make a picture of the baby you lost, using colours (crayons, perhaps, or fingerpaints). Don't worry about how 'artistic' it is. Do this until you have caught the right 'feel'. Place the picture where you can look at it over the next few days.

Keep a journal in which you jot down any sensations or feelings or dreams which might be connected with the lost baby. There are no rules for what you should feel. You don't need to censor what you write; this is for you alone.

The process of finding images may be gradual and irregular, akin to reverie or dreaming: time doesn't matter. One can take 'all the time in the world' to map the contours of the loss. Putting it into words or pictures reflects the woman back to herself, puts her at the centre of her experiences. Reading her journal or looking at her pictures can give her a sense of reality – 'realisation' – if there has been a lot of turmoil, or if her reaction has so far been superficial.

I Don't Have to Go it Alone

Most women probably find that their recovery cannot progress very far unless they are able to talk about their loss to other people. Mostly this happens informally or accidentally, without structures. Sharing experiences in this way is usually confirming and supportive, a great relief at getting it off one's chest. There may be great initial excitement and shared release when tears flow and hugs are given and got.

Sometimes, though, it does not fulfil all the needs a woman may have. She still may not feel afterwards that she has been really heard – particularly if the other woman or women also wanted to tell their stories. In order for her to hear herself (which is what it's about), she needs to be heard by someone whose undivided attention is directed at what she is really saying, with her face and body as well as her words. But the listener needs to be heard also, and unless there is some kind of agreement about this, 'sharing' our experiences may be more a matter of competing for available airspace or else of swallowing down what we feel for fear of talking too much.

> With your partner, decide who talks first. Each has ten minutes to talk while the other listens – it is important to share the time absolutely equally. The person listening takes responsibility for calling time, so the speaker's attention can be on herself. She is using this space to hear herself. The listener helps her do this by putting her attention in silence on the speaker. At the end of ten minutes, the listener gives feedback for the speaker from what she heard and observed. The listener and speaker then exchange roles.

The activity of structuring our talking, of making our needs more explicit, may feel uncomfortable, as it touches on anxieties like 'I don't deserve this attention' or 'I daren't expose my weaknesses to other women'. These anxieties themselves can be voiced and deprived of some of their negative power. Taking oneself seriously can be thought of as a skill that can be learnt by doing and by following each other's sample.

What About a Group?

This is how self-help groups – now a flourishing form of health-related activity in the UK – have often been started. Though the idea of creating one may sound daunting, in practice many of them have grown out of evening classes, mother and toddler clubs, meetings or friendship groups. Participating in self-help therapy over a length of time requires commitment and preparation, to be sure; one of the best books on the subject is *In Our Own Hands* by Sheila Ernst and Lucy Goodison,[1] which covers setting up, organising and sustaining a self-help therapy group as well as trouble-shooting possible problems. It provides substantial work-shop material through sample approaches – such as gestalt, co-counselling, psychodrama, encounter – to a variety of themes.

Self-help in a group can be a tremendously empowering activity, but if everyone is feeling uncertain to begin with, it may do to consider inviting an outsider, whether on a voluntary or paid basis, to lead the group, at least initially. Another strategy is for each member to take a turn at leading a session. This would entail responsibilities like starting the meeting, since people can be nervous about actually getting to work; negotiating an agenda of what each person wants to do during the meeting; time-keeping and bringing the session to a close. These are basic practices important to the running of a group and it may help if they are the responsibility of someone in particular.

When several women share their painful experiences there is likely to be turbulence – anger, fear, grief are explosively near the surface. If no one is an expert, how can anyone know what to do or how to cope? If they all get upset at once, who's going to sort it out? How can they deal with the differences between them cons-tructively? This is where clear guidelines are useful: the group is giving each woman permission to have and to express 'difficult' feelings. The group is there to help to contain these feelings, to allow them safe existence. The group is not there primarily to make judgements or give advice – each woman will have had plenty of both already, a lot of it from inside her own head. Women are often very good at hearing the smallest nuance of criticism, real or imaginary; it takes very little for most women to be deflected from attention to their own needs. The group's primary task is to establish a collective safety, to become, temporarily but un-conditionally, a loving environment for each of its members. Its main assumption is that each woman has good reason for her feelings. Members should not take responsibility for resolving each other's emotional problems: self-help is based on the premise that each person can, given permission, understand and heal herself. Of course this premise may not always hold good in a straightforward way – some people need specialised individual help or stronger intervention and a self-help group is not the most appropriate medium for this.

Usually the sense of a common enterprise builds quickly and collective self-confidence along with it. It may help to spend part of an early session drawing up a group contract which incorporates agreed goals. This can be reviewed every few weeks. Shifts in emphasis and direction can be monitored together so that each woman can have a say in what the group is doing overall, rather than changes 'just happening'. It may happen as the group gets established that issues arise which must somehow be dealt with. Class, race and sexuality are not baggage to be left in the hall while 'pure feelings' are all that's allowed in. Prejudices may masquerade as feelings; feelings may be profoundly shaped by women's experiences as members of an oppressed class or race. It is a truism, for instance, but more than ever true, not only that white middle-class women have better access to health care than black or working-class women, but also that the incidence of ante and postnatal complications, including miscarriage, is lower among better-off women. Some groups which have begun on a self-help basis have taken the campaigning road or have gone out into their communities to do health education work. Many groups success-fully combine strategies; 'going public' can build confidence and self-esteem, while working on one's own feelings can provide a sound basis for supporting other people and stimulating other groups.

What Am I Telling Myself

A woman's encounter with loss connects her powerfully with feelings of failure and guilt, with sometimes horrendously des-tructive messages from herself. Whether she works on her own, with a partner or in a group, she can learn to listen dispassionately to them. She may be able to recognise patterns from the past that got threaded into the event. 'You failed again', 'Why did it have to be me?', 'Nobody understands' are repetitious inner voices with the power of veto or sabotage which thrive on setbacks. Paradoxically, they also block out deeper pain and rage. They give a dubious security to our lives by confirming our anxieties. Letting them have their say is the first step in nullifying their power. Identifying them is the second.

> Take a cushion, put it in front of you and start talking to it. You are the voice with the message – say it loud and clear, whether it's 'You're making a fuss about nothing', 'You never were any good at anything', 'You didn't deserve that baby', or whatever. Go on until you've finished.

What we often do with internal conflicts is to try to get them to meet in the middle – this exercise acknowledges and acts

out the reality of that inner split. The next exercise belongs with
it.

Now it is the turn of the you that suffered and feels bad. Change
positions and put another cushion where you were just sitting, to
represent the 'voice'. Tell it what your feelings are now. Take this
time to express your grief and anger, uninterrupted by the voice
now it's not occupying all that space in your head. Go on until
you've finished.

Often this duo gets into a dialogue, turn and turn about. Eventually
the voice may be named and located, which may help to put it back
where it belongs. This can be a dramatic discovery, accompanied by
a great release of emotion. The voice may for many years have
prevented the woman from feeling her real feelings. Long ago,
perhaps as a very young child, she heard its message and it lodged in
her head as if it originated there. It was never safe to express her
feelings, even and especially to herself.

   One form of such a split may be about whether to undertake
therapy work: 'I don't need to go into all this', 'What's the use of
it?', 'It's all pretty self-indulgent, isn't it?' Some psychological and
psychiatric approaches echo parental we-know-better-than-you
voices; they are self-perpetuating and encourage dependence; they
may ultimately be reinforced by measures like hospitalisation,
enforced medication and loss of civil liberties. It seems healthy to
resist them. Resistance to all kinds of therapy, however, may be a
way of denying any vulnerability, when 'I don't need help anyway'
is equivalent to 'I'm frightened of anyone – including me – seeing
what a mess I am.' Such fear probably goes back to a time when it
was *not* safe for this person to be needy or in a mess. The first step,
of learning to feel one's feelings, however much the voices try to
push them out, may need to be taken whenever deeper or more
difficult feelings emerge.

What Are My Meanings?

Recovery comes in its own time, after some kind of descent into
mourning or depression. It is possible to choose this descent, to
abandon deliberately one's everyday self and meet the pain at a
deeper level. Pain is not a gift or a privilege or a spiritual status

symbol: it is not divine, it hurts. Women suffer a sufficient burden of unwanted, unsought hurts without going looking for more. But in inching a way through pain we have not sought we can progressively slough off the role of victim. And in meeting those hurtful or horrifying things with one's full intelligence it can often happen that a richer meaning for one's life is created.

What helpers/partners can do

1

Notice if the person is expressing something with her body, such as frowning, rocking, clenching her fists. Point this out gently. Suggest she exaggerates them, makes them consciously part of what's happening.

2

Notice if she is holding her breath or breathing shallowly. Encourage her, perhaps by placing your hand on her stomach or belly, to take deeper breaths. This may help her to contact feelings. Don't persist if she indicates she dislikes it.

3

Suggest she repeats a particular phrase – it might be something she has already said but passed over quickly. It must be simple and direct. You need to be very attentive for this.

4

Prompt her gently if she falls silent: 'What are you feeling now?'

5

If she wants physical contact, try supporting her from behind instead of giving her a hug. This enables her to carry on with what she's doing as well as to have someone close.

6

Do not rush in with advice, interpretation, opinion or your own feelings: make time for those later.

Prebirth loss has its own peculiar pains. It is not possible to be definitive about them, only to offer some trailers, such as:

Female biology, the biology of reproduction and its cycles, is problematic. Not inherently, as has been argued by gynaecologists and psychiatrists, but because of centuries of mistrust and fear of women's bodies. Women carry this mistrust inside them, it is passed on to them with their mothers' milk and their fathers' touch. Generations of this are not easily undone, not amenable to rational argument or legislation. One manifestation of this is that difficult menstruation and miscarriage sometimes run in the family; we inherit the pattern from our mothers and grandmothers as if it were genetic. To work on this unconscious patterning, to turn it round, requires an acceptance that much formative experience occurs before we are old enough to understand it or normally remember it (see Catherine's story on page 195).

Loss is one of those primal feelings. The loss of a baby, sad enough in itself, may trigger an earlier, unremembered loss and the present event may become instantly loaded with all that old and unexpressed grief too. The loss may be of a loved person who died or went away; or it may be the untimely loss of safety, innocence, childhood itself. The feelings may have been buried so deep and for so long that they may not have existed in any effective way in one's present life – until the event of miscarriage, abortion or ectopic pregnancy awakens them. It may be hard to locate their source, they may have the character of all-pervading unbearable tragedy at first.

Allow these feelings in, even though you may feel taken over by them. You can discover their source, but not by force. Try to give yourself lots of gentle love and attention. You have these feelings but you are not these feelings – there is more to you than them. Respect them. Ask them where they came from and what they have to tell you.

One of the commonest feelings involved in loss is *guilt*. Women blames themselves for what has happened. As Marilyn pointed out, women are damned either way: if they coddle and care for themselves while menstruating, pregnant or after a miscarriage, they're playing the part of the feeble female. If they cover up their vulnerability, they're suppressing their reality to fit in with someone else's demands – possibly with grave repercussions.

Some psychiatrists and gynaecologists like to imagine that miscarriage is a subconscious wish-fulfilment – she didn't want the baby. Theories like the 'blighted ovum', by contrast, envisage our

It is important to take these exercises slowly. Someone else could read them out with plenty of pauses so you can concentrate on what you're doing. Or you could make a tape for yourself.

Lie down somewhere comfortable. Start by relaxing in every part of your body, from your toes upwards. Breathe slowly and easily. You are going on a journey. Imagine yourself like Alice in Wonderland growing smaller and smaller . . . You are very tiny now. You are waiting at the entrance to your vagina. Notice how this place looks, how it smells, what colours you can see. Notice how you're feeling – maybe many feelings. Now leave them here outside. You can collect them later if you want to. All you need now is your ability to sense and observe. Begin to travel slowly inwards, through the lips. Go slowly, noting everything . . .

Now further in, into the tunnel. What's the journey like, how do you move, what can you see, hear, taste? . . .

Now ahead of you you can see the cervix. Think of it as a doorway. What does it look like, what kind of door is it? How do you get in? . . .

Now you are through. You are in the womb. Look all round you. See, hear, touch. Is there anything in particular to notice? Is there any place that feels hurt? If there is, go there and stay awhile. Let the place speak to you. What do you say in response? . . .

It is time to go on. Turning either left or right, travel into the passage which is the fallopian tube. How far can you get? What do you encounter? . . .

If you get to the end, you can see the ovary ahead of you. What does it look like, sound like? Spend as much time here as you need . . .

If you cannot get this far, what is stopping you? What do you have to do? Spend as much time here as you need . . .

Going deliberately as before, turn back and retrace your steps back into the womb. Do you see any differences? . . .

Take a last look and go out through the doorway. You have left the womb and are getting ready to emerge. Go carefully, let your senses guide you . . .

Now you are back on the threshold, about to re-enter the world. You will remember where you've been and what you did. Take a minute to rest and recover . . .

Now you are getting larger and larger. You are yourself again. In time, take a good cleansing breath and open your eyes.[2]

bodies as working in the best interests of the baby – but why was the ovum blighted in the first place? As if in answer to our feelings of powerlessness (see below), guilt holds us totally responsible for what happened. Our bodies have indeed sabotaged our conscious wishes, but how and why? Because we're bad, comes the answer. Acquiring information about miscarriage and ectopic pregnancy helps: it's not just me, and it wasn't because I went to the party/moved the wardrobe/masturbated when I was a young girl. (See Part Two.)

It can also help to give those voices their say, again with the aid of a cushion. Often it turns out that they are saying that to be a proper mother, deserving a healthy baby, you must observe strict limits. You must not work too hard or play too hard – your life must not be your own. This covert instruction needs a great deal of winkling out. It is not at all the same as the instruction to take good care of oneself, though it may borrow the other's clothes.

However, for some women, an exploration of the deep connections between mind and body may reveal an ambivalence about pregnancy and motherhood that expresses itself through the miscarriage. I came to the realisation a few months after my miscarriage that pregnancy had been altogether too frightening for me; I was not, as I thought, ready for it. Amongst the grief and rage I felt, there was a small sense of deliverance. I cannot now regard the miscarriage as coincidental. However, this kind of connection is for the individual woman to make; such knowledge, if it comes, belongs entirely to her. In any case, such is the oppression accompanying the reality of motherhood that a woman's ambivalent reaction to becoming a mother would be remarkable for its absence.

Loss may be attended by feelings of *powerlessness* on top of guilt: a woman may feel unable to initiate or direct, unable to do anything but react impulsively. Powerlessness is real – its effects are felt with differing intensity in different circumstances. Institutional power is out there staring us in the face and slapping us down, and therapy doesn't change power relations.

But how a woman relates to authority figures, some of whom have real power and some only illusory power over her, *can* be explored through therapy. She may be giving up her power so she feels powerless when she is not – or not as much as she feels. If, for instance, the medical professionals behaved unsympathetically during her miscarriage, she may have reacted to them in such a way as to lock herself more firmly into their labelling process – thus depriving herself further of what she needed. This is a double bind – to get what she wants, it seems a woman has to be 'a good girl' and play the game their way. Yet it is important to realise that some forms of confrontation do more harm to us as individuals than to the institutions which hurt us. Unsuccessful confrontation confirms those feelings of 'I'm no good', 'I don't deserve to be treated well', 'Nobody cares about me'. We need to recognise whose ground we are on. If we are away from home, so to speak, we can hardly hope to win if we up the stakes.

Yet negotiating rather than confronting, being assertive rather than aggressive or defensive, has to be from a position of felt strength. If the other person triggers unresolved feelings of powerlessness in us, we cannot negotiate, we can only yield or rebel like a child.

> Play out the scene with the doctor or nurse. Put them 'on a cushion' or ask your partner to adopt the role. Recreate the scene as it happened. Were your words really addressed to someone else in your life? What do you wish you had said instead? (Remember that this realisation of yours does not absolve the doctor and nurse of their behaviour.)

Pain and blood and the sense of physical powerlessness they induce accompany all prebirth loss, sometimes to a frightening extent. Many women feel totally out of control of their bodies. Giving birth, even in an early miscarriage, involves labour. Labour is more painful if fear is also present. None of the women who wrote for this book found their pain 'a slight cramp' as some text books describe it. Ectopic pregnancy is often diagnosed by the onset of severe pain. Add to this the possible pain of surgical intervention, and pain can seem at the heart of the experience. Perhaps it needn't be like this, as Helen Gould suggests (see pp. 151–2). But usually women do not receive ideal medical co-operation for handling their pain and are left with consequent self-doubt about being able to cope with pain. The meaning of the pain is somehow taken from them, as also happens too often in labour and delivery of a live baby.

The bleeding which preceded losing the baby may have been heavy and frightening. When a woman's monthly bleeding returns, not only is this a sign of not having conceived but also a vivid reminder of the death of her baby and the danger to herself. In short, many women suffer a great deal of distress on a physical level. It usually becomes just a memory, but it can leave a woman distrustful of her body, vulnerable to its power to hurt.

Women have been made to digest a toxic stodge of irrational fears about the female body, particularly about menstruation and blood – the curse. But with the growth of modern feminism, many have discovered a sense of pleasure and power in menstruation, a developing awareness of psychic inspiration as well as physical–emotional ebbs and flows. *The Wise Wound* by Peter Redgrove and Penelope Shuttle[3] was a pioneering book in this field.

Make sure you are feeling safe in your present environment; have someone with you. Slowly let yourself go back to the shock of when you started bleeding or having severe pain. Let yourself realise again that you might lose your baby. Feel your fear . . .

Let your body tremble or shake; let out its moans or cries . . . When you have had enough, come back to the present. Feel your health and strength flow back. Say, 'I am alive and well. I have health and strength in me' . . .

Look after yourself well for the rest of the day.

Contradictory feelings about *sexuality* may add to a woman's sense of 'badness'. One of the accusing voices may be saying, 'And you shouldn't have had sex – that's what caused the miscarriage.' On the one hand, society says that sex is for making babies. On the other hand, it says that good mothers don't have sex, though being sexy is what makes a woman desirable. You can't have sex and be a good mother; you can't deny sex and be a desirable woman.

Try saying out loud, 'Sex is about . . .' List the thoughts and images that occur to you.

Then say, 'My sexuality is about . . .'

Finally, say, 'Motherhood is about . . .

Compare all three lists. Do the first and third lists leave enough room for what's in the second?

At another level, sex is about intimacy. After prebirth loss a woman may react vehemently against sex or be driven by yearnings for it.

She may need to look at how much sexuality for her and her sexual partner is an expression of or a substitute for affection and nurturance. If she feels her partner was insufficiently sympathetic, couldn't or wouldn't share her grief, she may not feel like making her body open, particularly in a way which could render her vulnerable to pregnancy and miscarriage (or abortion) again. Or she may want a tangible demonstration of love, the reassurance that she's not a freak.

Or she may want to get pregnant again as soon as possible to prove she can do it. She may want to be filled up again, to feel the emptiness assuaged. Sex at the best of times is a conduit for so much wordless traffic between people.

Questions worth asking in relation to sex, affection and intimacy are:

How well do I take in the good things in my life?

How well do I keep out the bad things?

Where are my boundaries and how do I make others aware of them?

How do I ask for, and get, what I need?

What does sex mean for me?

Giving Birth to Myself?

Doing therapy is not a substitute for having a baby. Writing a book or painting a picture is not a substitute for having a baby. Perhaps nothing can ever take the place of the baby we lost. But women are pressurised into diverting their entire creativity into procreation. At some stage in her recovery, a woman may need to look at what 'baby' means. Powerful evocations may surface: there is, perhaps, a part of her that needs to be born, to see the light of day. Therapy will not decide whether she should try to make another baby, but it can illuminate her reasons for doing so and at the same time release more of her creativity in other areas.

Can I Let Go?

As Mary Anne says, most of us need to go through a period of mourning for what we have lost, devising rituals, performing

Talk to your baby. Use a small soft cushion or anything else that has a 'baby' feel. Hold it close and say:

I wanted you because . . .

What you mean to me is . . .

The place you have in my life is . . .
The colour of that place is . . .
The sound of that place is . . .
The name of that place is . . .

Keep a journal of your dreams.

symbolic burials, commemorating anniversaries. We should not underestimate the healing power of these things. Death is a mystery with which we may need to come to terms each time it happens. The snuffing out of the life-spark seems to demand something from us. In time, most of us reach the point where we can let go of the experience. Hanging on is natural – it takes time to incorporate what we've learnt. We may also hang on because we feel guilty that a part of us already wants to go on with life; or because we are anxious that people will expect us to get back to normal. An indication that it is time to let the experience drop back into the general pattern of one's life is a sense of boredom with it. One woman said she couldn't bear to read her account again – not because it was too painful, but because it had nothing more to say to her.

Concluding Thoughts

It is true that in the 1990s self-help therapies no longer appeal only to a small minority, nor are they viewed with undifferentiated suspicion. There is apparently a wealth of resources and a huge variety of help and support available. The problem is rather the substitution of 'self-help' for a well-funded and properly resourced National Health Service, so that having access to those resources may depend more and more on having the money to buy them or living in an area where there are still cheap venues for hire, well-stocked libraries, a robust community health policy with expert back-up if you need it. It is not just a question of supporting self-help as a strategy in healing, which of course it is; we need at the same time to understand and combat the ways in which the health-care market robs women of control over the resources for (as well as the meanings of) the events in their biological lives in the guise of giving us more so-called choice.

My place

Permission to depart please,
And return to the sea of
perpetual peace.
My place/nta.
The womb of my own.
My mother.
My cuntry.

Lindsay James

Life Before Birth:
An Inside Story

Lindsay James

I am the mother of four children, two young adults in their twenties and two teenagers. I have never had a miscarriage myself, but I am someone who survived the threatened miscarriage my mother had when she was pregnant with me. I am someone who as a foetus of about four months was almost 'spontaneously aborted'. I nearly died, but I didn't. I survived, both to my mother's and my own relief.

I have acquired my understanding about the significance of prebirth experience both professionally as a psychotherapist working with women and men on what I regard as the adult symptoms of intra-uterine trauma, and personally as a 'patient' in psychoanalysis.

I think of 'my miscarriage' as a terrible, traumatic experience which subsequently shaped my whole life, although I was unaware of its power and influence over me until, approaching the age of 40, the pain – the emotional legacy of that prebirth experience – became so unbearable that really I was forced to let go of it. This I did, gradually, over a period of several years through therapy.

This process has given me a unique perspective on myself both as a daughter, and as a mother: and some knowledge of what I think are the needs of both mothers and babies during pregnancy, particularly in relation to miscarriage or threatened miscarriage. Here I weave my 'inside story' together with some insights I have had about mothering as a result of having uncovered the occluded experience of surviving a miscarriage. I can imagine that this will have meaning for mothers who have lost or who will in the future lose their babies through miscarriage and abortion, and also for mothers whose babies survived threatened miscarriages or attempted abortions. I can also imagine it speaking to mothers who want to find ways of being close to their babies from conception onwards, and to adults who themselves survived a threatened miscarriage (or even an attempted abortion) before their birth.

For many people, the notion that it is possible to have been influenced 'psychologically' while in the womb and then to have any 'memory' of this will be regarded as ridiculous. But that is only, I think, because people are disconnected from this experience and because it is not 'remembered' in a conventional – i.e. conscious – way, so it is not known and acknowledged generally in the medical, psychology or psychiatric professions. Other forms of memory – the subconscious, intuition and feelings – are not accorded the same status and value as rational, intellectual, objective, empirical thought. So the whole period of prebirth life, birth itself, and to some extent infancy too, are rarely taken into account meaningfully and appropriately as the life experience of an individual.

The real loss – in the 'hidden loss' this book is about – is the fact that this whole dimension of experience is largely 'hidden' and unacknowledged. That has begun to change with the publication of medical and psychoanalytic work on 'the aware baby'[1], 'the secret life of the unborn child'[2], 'how to overcome pre-natal trauma'[3], on being born[4], and, more recently, observational studies of the life of the foetus before birth and its effects on the psychology and behaviour of the child after birth[5].

My own personal and professional experience has convinced me that there is everything to gain from connecting both with our selves and our prebirth experience, and with our babies before they are born. There are, however, some very real dangers in doing so: for 'feminism' and for the lives of women generally. This is because women's wombs and 'the foetus' have been appropriated now by religious fundamentalism and its 'right to life' ideology. This operates effectively (and also, I think, intentionally) as another mechanism of the social control of women and their bodies. There is the risk, therefore, that acknowledging and exploring our experience as mothers – and the experience of our children – from conception onwards will provide 'the patriarchs' with material that can be used to attack feminism and to further subordinate women. For individual women and their pro-abortion, 'women's right to choose' allies, this can be and has been literally a life or death matter. It is not lightly, therefore, that I share my 'inside story.'

An Experiential Account

I began my life in September 1942 in Scotland where I was conceived in the middle of the Second World War when my father was home on leave. I might have deduced the date of my conception from the fact that I was born in June 1943, had I ever thought the date of my conception was of anything but academic interest. Now I count my life from the beginning: it's the only way I have been able to account for how I came to be as I was, as I am. This is what I have come to 'remember' and to 'reconstruct' of my first nine months.

When I was about four months old (dating from my conception, or five months, counting back from my birth) I was nearly miscarried or 'spontaneously aborted' (in medical terminology). I have always known this because my mother would tell the story of how she had started bleeding in about the fourth month of her (our) pregnancy; of how she had gone immediately to bed and stayed there on the advice of her doctor that bed rest was all that she could do to prevent a possible miscarriage. The obstetrician who attended my birth had then apparently commented to her, after my birth, about the amount of scar tissue there was in the (my) placenta, how it was a 'miracle' I had survived: that if she had not taken such drastic steps to look after herself (and me), I would almost certainly have been miscarried (a word we use that would have meant my death). Hearing the story always makes me feel how much wanted and how much loved I had been – and how lucky to be alive.

From my mother's point of view, I was a wanted baby and a planned pregnancy. My conception was a conscious decision, not an accident. My parents had moved to Glasgow from Dundee when my father had taken up a job as a GP after they had married in 1941, and shortly thereafter my father had been called up. He was, in fact, to die in the war and sadly I was never to know him. My mother's life at this time was extremely stressful. When I was born, she was living on her own, separated from my father and her family, in a strange city during war time. In spite of this, my mother and I were very happy with our coexistence in the first four months of 'our' pregnancy.

From my point of view, I think my first four months were a time of well-being, and being well. I have a sense of how I must have been at one with myself and my world – my womb, and my mother. Secure, complete and whole at each stage of my development from my conception onwards. Self-aware, self-satisfied – with a 'self'. Creative and content to be just as I was at whatever stage of development I was at (see Appendix 4). Alive – and aware of it in every fibre of my growing self.

What I believe happened next was that suddenly – terribly, horribly, awfully suddenly – I started to slip away. I was terrified. Utterly terrified, in a panic. Bewildered, confused. It was as if I couldn't breathe, as if I was gasping for breath. Rigid. I'd been lying there, curled up, very contented, thinking: 'How wonderful it is to be alive'. Suddenly: 'Hey, what's happening? Hang on . . .' Confusion. Next thought: 'Help'. Then nothing. No thoughts, I couldn't think. Blank. I was frozen with fear, quite paralysed with it, rigid. Every bit of my being was focused on surviving. I 'held my breath'. Didn't move, didn't breathe. Just what people do at any age when they are frightened and in danger. Sudden adrenalin. I kept very still, didn't move a muscle, held my breath. And survived – to my present age of 45 (counting from my birth) or 46 (dating from my conception).

Images I have now, of what happened to me then: my life-support system coming unplugged, the vessels of my placenta one by one pulling out, the gradual dawning realisation of what was happening: the actual disintegrating of my life-support system and the feeling, the fear of my *own* imminent disintegration – of death. The fear of falling out of the womb: like being in an airplane with the fear of falling out of the sky.

Connecting the Present with the Past

For me, it was a fear of flying that took me into therapy initially and began my journey back to my beginnings. Apart from my mother's story about 'her' miscarriage, I was unaware of what had happened to me and I was most certainly unaware of any connections between my fear of flying and my miscarriage. What I was to discover over the next four years were what I came to understand to be very direct connections between that event and this fear, plus many other fears (including claustrophobia) and all the other ways my life had always been difficult. The process of these discoveries is a story for another place, but I will make a brief summary of the 'personality' or 'psychological symptoms' that originated from that prebirth experience: for other adults who might recognise these in themselves and have always wondered how they might have come to be as they are, or for parents who might recognise these in their children and have always been bewildered by certain behaviours. For knowing now what happened to me then, I feel that I can understand life patterns and behaviours that previously had been a source of confusion and pain.

The fear of dying, then, stayed with me. I spent the next 40 years of my life waiting – minute by minute – to die. Literally not a day of my life passed without my worrying about my sudden and imminent death. I tried to analyse it and locate the origins of the fear in certain childhood experiences and adolescent losses. Although I had not had a 'happy' childhood there was nothing that could really account for the amount of my fear. Now that I know about my own near-death in the womb – now that I am connected with this experience as a part of my life – the fear I have always lived with, the terror, seems an appropriate and reasonable reaction to what happened then.

Physically, I have always been rigid and tense, especially in my back and shoulders. I have also been an 'anxious' person: anxiety etched on my face like a mask. You could see it, if you could see beyond the 'grin' of terror that I also wore most of my life, and which people often mistook for friendliness. I used to joke about the constant anxiety: 'I've been like this since before I was born'. Little did I know! The anxiety now seems to have been a natural response to waiting daily for sudden death: the clip in the back of the neck, the stab in the back.

The pattern of periods in my life of acute anxiety is now apparent: most acute at times of major rejections – like leaving home, losing a job, losing a husband. Rejection by anyone – but especially women – has always been a source of great terror to me. Even the smallest rejections have seemed like a threat of death, particularly if I have dared to 'trust'. Trusting anyone – really trusting – has been 'more than my life was worth': dangerous. Any betrayals of the little bits of trust I have allowed myself have been utter devastations. Angry women terrify me. All of this makes sense, of course, if you appreciate the position of a four month foetus: naturally trusting and dependent and then faced with the ultimate rejection by the one person it has to rely on totally for survival: its mother, that woman.

I've always been an angry person. Much of my anger has been directed at my mother, probably from the time of my birth. This must have been very bewildering for her. I do distinctly 'remember' what a great relief it was to get out of that place – that womb that for me felt like a tomb. Safety at last. I have an image of myself as completely self-reliant from the moment I was born: feeding myself, changing my own nappies. Of course this was never true, but it will have felt that I'd had to rely on myself solely, *on my own*, for my survival in the womb and I obviously decided then that self-reliance was the only way to survive. I've often prided myself on my 'independence', and been praised for it. A more appropriate word for this would have been isolation: it has been very lonely.

My feelings of worthlessness have always been immeasurable,

quite outrageously out of proportion to my worth and how it has been validated by *everyone* in my life, quite without exception. However much I have been loved – and I have most certainly been enormously well-loved and appreciated – the overwhelming feelings have been of being utterly unloved, and unlovable. My desperation to be loved has been a life or death matter: sending out messages of 'please like me', and seeking out love and approval. Grateful for morsels of attention. Very humiliating.

I definitely never felt that I deserved to be alive, that I had any right to be here on earth. The very idea used to make me laugh. Everyone – everything – was infinitely more important than me. If it would really do the world a favour, I would gladly have died.

How could I, given what had happened, really believe that I was lovable and worthy of being loved? The message I must have got then was of being loved for a while by someone (my mother) who had a change of heart and then wanted to get rid of me. Without any information to the contrary I must have concluded that there was 'something wrong with me'. Since then, in relationships, I have always wondered what people saw in me in the first place and then, if they were persistent enough to make a relationship, waited (anxiously) until they discovered the dreadful secret (whatever it is, because I've never known) of why my mother wanted 'to get rid of me'. Such terrible irony, of course, that this was never my mother's intention, and from her point of view, wasn't what happened at all; but from my point of view I don't think I could have known otherwise and would have internalised the plain, simple fact that (for some reason) I wasn't wanted. Babies who survive attempted abortions have similar feelings too, I think, but no knowledge of the circumstances – the stresses and pressures – that will have forced their mothers to attempt abortion.

Some of the 'survival strategies' – the legacy of that early life-threat – are regarded as extremely socially acceptable, even desirable. I'm a 'doer', an 'organiser', a high-achiever in every aspect of my life. I've prided myself on being a 'superwoman': I've been praised for it. Always busy. Very productive. 'How do you do it?' people often ask in admiration. But I *have* to keep functioning. It's a compulsion, not a choice. Keep moving in order not to feel the *unbearable* feeling of being still – and being reminded of the stillness in the womb. Not daring to move, for fear of falling out, of dying: the terror, anything but the terror.

In reality, there is nothing attractive about living at a literally *killing* pace: it's a struggle, it's exhausting. As is the fear, the isolation, the desperation to be loved and the inability to feel love and to feel lovable. To be such a 'divided self' – so divided, so disconnected from your self, your essence, your very existence – is a dreadful, daily, grinding, exhausting struggle.

Then there is the constant struggle to *think* through the legacy of confusion from that early incident, accident. I have always found it difficult to think in any situation I regarded as important. The more important, the nearer to life or death it seemed, the greater the panic. Then blank. The panic rising from my stomach up through my chest, into my throat and finally into my brain. And I'd be paralysed. But not before it stopped my breath, choked me, left me gasping. My mind blank, thoughts fragmented, confusion, and I would act stupidly or not at all. A struggle to breathe. A struggle to think. Just like way back, in the womb.

I smoked almost as soon as I could, using cigarettes to keep the fear at bay, so I could think, and breathe. Or so it felt, for in reality smoking stops you breathing and though it makes you 'feel better', it actually kills you. But, if you are a survivor of this kind of prebirth trauma, you 'feel so awful' all your life, you'd do almost anything to 'feel better'. You'll look for any relief to the 'depression': to the struggle of 'holding on for dear life' you've been doing almost from the beginning.

Connecting the Experiential and the Empirical

Since first writing in this way about my experience in 1989, in the first edition of *Hidden Loss*, I found in Piontelli's *From Fetus to Child*, in 1992, a similar account of the effects of a threatened miscarriage on a foetus as observed before birth by means of ultrasound and subsequently during and after the birth on the personality and behaviour of the infant and the child in its first three years of life. Observed ultrasonically at the twentieth week, the foetus is described by the doctor as 'moving a lot and exploring a lot', as 'definitely a lively one', as 'a very active child': swallowing, yawning, scratching its ears, touching its chin and feet and chest, kicking against the uterine wall, somersaulting and curling up. It is also observed as 'squashing the placenta', 'dipping its nose in the placenta', its 'lips in contact with the placenta', 'trying to pull the placenta towards itself', and as 'trying to detach the placenta'. At one point, the doctor becomes anxious and says, with reference to the foetus and the placenta: 'you be careful, stop doing it, it is dangerous you know, you could be detaching it.'

In the days following this ultrasonic observation, the pregnant woman started bleeding heavily, denoting a detaching of the placenta and a probable miscarriage. The woman was ordered absolute rest for awhile and given drugs to prevent a miscarriage. Pinotelli described the effect on Pina (the name given to the child when she was born) as being 'dramatic': 'during the third ultrasonic observation (in the thirtieth week) she seemed to have lost all her appetite and her movement. She . . . was tightly crouched in a corner of the womb and completely immobile'[6]. Pina stayed in this position for the remainder of the pregnancy and was delivered by Caesarean. The doctor was struck by the fact that the baby 'seemed greatly relieved to be out' and described her as a 'vivacious and alert child'. One of her feet, however, due to malposition in utero had to be put in plaster for several months. Pinotelli observed the child at two months and commented on her alertness and the amount of her movement, but also described her as a 'rather tense child' and observed 'many fears, particularly of not being held securely and of falling.' The mother described her daughter as 'keeping everything under control with her eyes'.

The child suffered from 'acute claustrophobic anxieties' in confined places, fear of falling and not being held securely. She was also 'frightened of being left alone in a void and could not bear silence'. She would 'react to people or events with great, mounting excitement' which 'very soon' would turn into 'fear and crying and her explorations into tragedy'[7]. She was a very 'precocious child who desperately seemed to want to grow up fast'. She began to talk and crawl by 8 months, by 13 months she could walk and 'was talking like a much older child'. Observed then, at the age of three years, she 'looked and behaved as if she were older than her age' and did 'everything for herself'. Piontelli observed as characteristics of Pina's personality, a 'persisting tendency towards vigorous activity, almost hyperactivity, accompanied or followed by fear of disaster and tragedy'[8].

Although it was not my personal experience, I have treated adults who have recovered memories of having lost a twin in utero, and of being a 'single surviving twin'. In one account, a client has described her earliest memory of a time when she had a twin brother while she was in the womb. She described the 'sense of complete love, trust, relaxation, communication and well-being that they shared'. She then described 'a cord somehow being caught in his mouth' so that she 'was losing oxygen'. She described 'starting to float backwards' and 'to pass out' and 'as a reflex motion, kicking him in the head'. She then perceived 'a reddish tint to the amniotic fluid' followed by 'vivid images of his body decaying and disintegrating and then disappearing' and her search for him, leaving her with 'tremendous anxiety, devastation, grief, loneliness and confusion.' Another client described how being born with this kind of incident behind you 'makes you feel like you've lived a hundred years', how she keeps looking for her lost twin everywhere, and seeking people 'just like me' to be close to. Research on adult twins who lost their twin at different times of life found a 'significant correlation [in effects] for twins who lost their twin before six months'[9]. They were sometimes blamed by parents for the death of their twin. One mother accused her ten-year-old daughter of 'having caused her twin to be dismembered before birth'. Twins who were told in childhood that they had lost a twin at birth, confirmed 'how this information made "sense" of feelings that they had previously experienced which had seemed mysterious'[10].

Acknowledging Life Before Birth

What is to be gained from looking squarely at so much anxiety and struggle? For myself, finding the resources through therapy to face the fear finally enabled me to *feel* some of the pain that had been so unbearable then, but which *was* bearable (just) now that I am an adult and not a four month foetus, and to 'let go' at last of much of the fear and isolation and struggle I have just described. Going through this process has given me 'my life back' (the words that always come to mind), has enabled me to give up some of the compulsive and addictive behaviours (including smoking) and to replace them with real connections with myself and others, satisfying and secure relationships, peace, security, creativity and work that I choose to do.

Discovering the *reasons* for my deeply troubled and tormented existence has made the profoundest difference, because now I think I know why I was so damaged, why my life was so difficult, why my relationships were so fraught, and I no longer have a need to blame myself or to blame my mother or to blame anyone or anything else. I no longer need to be a 'victim'.

It has made me closer to and more understanding of my mother and more understanding as a mother of what has been hard for my children and why. For it is quite clear to me now that they – and everyone else in the world too – were *experiencing* their lives before they were born and that they too have some of this legacy to live with and to let go of. With the knowledge I now have, and especially with the very *acknowledgement* of their experience, I am in a position and I have the power to assist in the process of freeing people from the effects of this trauma, both at the time it may be taking place and also in retrospect.

Good Mothering from Conception Onwards

Every woman should have the right and the opportunity to choose whether or not to have a baby at all at any time in her life. Ideally that choice should come without pressure (i.e. the conditioning that to be a full, complete, successful or 'real' woman, you need to be a mother) or sanction (which labels the child 'free' as child 'less'). Ideally, that choice should be able to be made reliably in advance of pregnancy, with simple, safe and effective contraception. But these 'choices' are often not available so it is essential that women have the right to choose whether or not to have children even after they become pregnant – through abortion. Furthermore women should be able to make this choice and take this course of action without feelings of guilt, for in the absence of other freedoms, abortion is a freedom of choice that we require, and indeed it *can* free us of an unwanted or otherwise impossible pregnancy. At the same time, women should not have to pretend that abortion is a course of action they would choose if they had real freedom of choice with regard to getting pregnant and becoming a mother.

Individual women – in these circumstances – are blameless and are, in fact, always doing their very best, taking everything into account. It is important to acknowledge and to accept this as women in relation to pregnancy: whether it is a 'wanted' or 'unwanted' pregnancy, whether it involves a threatened miscarriage or attempted abortion, whether it ends in actual miscarriage or actual abortion, whether it continues to childbirth and child-rearing.

It is also possible to take steps to alleviate the negative effects on those who are experiencing or who have experienced their mother's miscarriage or attempt to abort them. I believe it would have made a difference to me as a foetus to have had *a genuine acknowledgement of my existence*: that *I was there and experiencing what was happening*. This would have required my mother to establish that *connection* with me: either by communicating inside, directing her thoughts and feelings to me inwardly and/or by talking to me out loud. What I needed to hear was *information about what was happening: the truth.* So I needed to hear:

that we are experiencing a threatened miscarriage and what that involved to the best of her knowledge

that *she* didn't know why

that *she* felt frightened and confused and isolated and lonely

that my life was at risk for some reason she did not just then have control over

that she was doing her best to save me

that she knew I was *also* struggling to save myself and that I would be feeling frightened and hurt

that she wanted me to live and that she knew I wanted to live, but that if in the circumstances *I* couldn't make it, that *we* didn't have enough resources to enable me to survive, that it was okay to fail in the struggle to survive and therefore to die

that my life was precious to her and would have been valuable and valued even if it had been very short and had ended then and there

that if I survived the miscarriage she would understand what I had been through and would give me all the attention I needed to recover after my birth

that she loved me and thought I was lovable.

I believe that, for me, the foetus, this would have made an enormous difference and would have significantly lessened the traumas of that experience. Pinotelli, for example, describes Pina as being 'helped by her understanding and very observant mother (and grandmother) to overcome many of the terrors belonging to her past. Contrary to her original plans, her mother waited well into spring before considering going back to work, and was always very attentive to soothe Pina and comfort her whenever her fears of falling or her claustrophic anxieties seemed to overwhelm her'[11].

I actually think that communication like this between mothers and babies in the *normal* course of a pregnancy would vastly improve the quality of life of any baby before it is born and the quality of the relationship between mother and child. The key issues are: *acknowledgement* (of the baby's existence, of a trauma if and when it is occurring, and of the pain and suffering it will be causing); *information* (about what is happening, day to day, and particularly at the time of the trauma); *connection* (between the two 'people' living in the same body, establishing and developing that relationship).

In the case of a woman whose circumstances force her to have an abortion, I think this form of communication with her baby is vitally important for herself as well as the baby. It could easily just take the form of focusing one's attention on the 'foetus', acknowledging its existence, at whatever stage of development it may be, explaining the circumstances that are bringing about a decision to have an abortion, communicating that its life has nevertheless been valuable and valued and that it is loved, or that she cares about it and is sorry to have to 'choose' abortion. This kind of connection is a real and positive alternative to the self-alienating disconnection we are forced to endure in order not to 'feel guilt'. If we know, and are also told, that we have nothing to feel guilty about, that we are doing the very best we can, taking all circumstances into account, then we can be freed to have this kind of connection with our bodies, our babies, our selves. And it opens up the opportunity to grieve as well – for the loss of a baby through miscarriage or abortion.

Medical interventions are sometimes necessary and helpful to save a threatened pregnancy: ultrasound scans, sometimes X-rays, amniocentesis, stitching the cervix under anaesthetic, and so forth. Communicating with our babies during these procedures can again make 'all the difference': acknowledging the baby's existence and *its* experience of the procedure; imagining and empathising with the baby's experience; giving information about what is going on; providing reassurance; communicating love.

Valerie describes how she explained to her baby (now daughter Laura) what would happen when they had an anaesthetic early in their pregnancy: how they would feel drugged and go temporarily unconscious, but then come awake again and perhaps feel a bit foggy, but would cope and survive, even though it might feel weird and scary. I think this kind of communication matters to both mothers and babies. If there's no 'proof that it helps', there is also no evidence that it causes 'harm' – and there is unlikely to be, because what harm could it possibly cause? Communicating like this would probably be regarded as common sense, if we had the sense to extend our imagination back a bit from the moment of birth when we can see a fully formed and 'feeling' and/or experiencing infant, and recognise that the infant was before the birth just as s/he is after the birth: a complete human being. And then to extend the imagination back, stage by stage from birth to conception, recognising the 'completeness' of the human being (or the potential human being) at whatever stage, whether a cluster of cells or with developing feet, fingers, features, heart, lungs, nervous system (see Appendix 4).

The point is *not* whether the foetus has a brain or an intellect or touch or smell or the ability to feel pain (though there is evidence that it does) or whether it is a 'viable life', but simply that it is completely alive in whatever way is appropriate at each stage of development and *experiencing itself* in whatever ways it can and will do at each stage. It exists (in whatever form) and its experiences (whatever they are) are its life; and, if and when it is born and grows through childhood to adulthood, these experiences will always be part of its life, part of what makes it who and how it is. In that sense the disconnection and lack of acknowledgement of this prebirth part of our lives effectively robs us of an important part of our lives and experience. That in itself is a loss – a grievous loss in my view. It causes us to lose part of our relationship (connection) with our selves, and part of our relationship with our mothers and our children. It is an unnecessary loss because it is possible to re-claim this experience.

Recovering from Early Hurts

The last point is to address again, from a slightly different angle, the process of recovering from prebirth traumas. If you are the mother and you've lost your baby through miscarriage or abortion, you need to grieve in the different ways that people experience grief and bereavement.

If you have children who have survived any kind of prebirth trauma, they too will benefit from being able to deal with some of the effects of their trauma and can best be 'treated' as if they were suffering from post-traumatic stress syndrome. Providing this additional care can be very hard on mothers who are already doing too much in too much isolation and suffering a lot of exhaustion. But to recognise that this is an essential part of the recovery or healing process can help: knowing that it is information, re-assurance and just good, patient attention that the baby needs.

The truth of the matter is, however, that *everyone* would benefit from having their prebirth existence acknowledged and attention paid to their prebirth experiences both before and after their birth;

because the good experiences prior to birth are part of each person's life story and everyone will also have had unpleasant or painful experiences (even if they haven't experienced a life-or-death trauma), because the world includes many unpleasant and painful things which will inevitably influence pregnant women and through them their developing babies. No one is immune from prebirth hurt or harm.

If you are an adult who recognises yourself to be a survivor of prebirth trauma such as threatened miscarriage or attempted abortion, you would probably find it helpful to use one of a number of possible 'therapeutic resources' to re-connect with the experiences you had then and to access the emotional release you need and no doubt long for. There are many forms of counselling and therapy available now and ways to facilitate healing. Lesley writes about some of the therapies and techniques available.

The first step, however, is to become sensitive to the experience of life before birth for both mothers and babies.

Part Five:
Appendices

1
References

Inside Stories

Mary Anne's Story
1 As explained on p. 96, the symptoms for these conditions can be similar.

Valerie's Story
1 It is interesting that this word is not the equivalent of 'nursing' and in fact is a pejorative term, meaning to adulterate or tamper with.
2 By 1995, foetuses as young as 21 or 22 weeks have survived.

Sheila's Story
1 Boston Women's Health Collective, *Our Bodies, Ourselves* Penguin, 1978, p. 501. This book was one of the very few women's health books available at the time. The almost complete absence of information was even more noticeable than in a non-feminist publication.

Marilyn's Story
1 This drug was probably HCG (human chorionic gonadotrophin). There is no proven benefit in its use in this situation but neither can the drug do any harm.

Ann's Story
1 Boston Women's Health Collective, *Our Bodies, Ourselves*, Penguin, 1978.

Helen's Story
1 Eggs can travel from one ovary across to the opposite fallopian tube if the tube on the same side has been removed (see p. 105). The literature on rates of successful pregnancy following miscarriage or ectopic pregnancy is confusing, as so much depends on individual circumstances. However, given the combination of Helen's age and the fact that having an ectopic pregnancy does increase the chance of another one (see p. 94), her chances of a safe pregnancy would probably be less than 50 per cent.

2 An 'in vitro' programme offers a couple the chance of fertilisation and hopefully conception outside the womb. If one or more eggs is fertilised, it is returned to the womb for growth and nurturance.

Part Two: Medical Viewpoints

1 The Miscarriage Association's Newsletter, Spring 1986.

Part Three: The Key Issues

1 Alice Lovell, *New Society*, 4 August 1983, p. 167.
2 See Lesley Saunders, 'Sex and Childbirth', in S. Cartledge and J. Ryan (eds.), *Sex and Love: New Thoughts on Old Contradictions*, The Women's Press, 1983.
3 J. Le Grand, 'Quasi-markets and Social Policy', in *The Economic Journal*, 101, 1991, pp. 1256–67.
4 Libby Purves, *How Not to be a Perfect Mother*, Fontana, 1986, p. 22.
5 Boston Women's Health Collective, *Our Bodies, Ourselves*, Penguin, 1978.
6 Chris Pope, *Peace News*, 20 February 1976.
7 Eileen Fairweather, 'The Feelings Behind the Slogans', in *Spare Rib*, 87, October 1979; reprinted in *No Turning Back*, Feminist Anthology Collective (ed.), The Women's Press, 1981, pp. 30, 31.
8 See Lynda Rajan, '"Not Just Me Dreaming". Parents Mourning Pregnancy Loss', in *Health Visitor*, vol. 65 (10), 1992, pp. 354–7; 'Social Isolation and Support in Pregnancy Loss; in Health Visitor, vol. 67(3), 1994, pp. 97–101; and Ann Oakley and Lynda Rajan, 'No Pills for Heartache: The Importance of Social Support for Women Who Suffer Pregnancy Loss', in *Journal of Reproduction and Infant Psychology*, vol. 11, 1993, pp. 75–87.

Part Four: Coming Through and Going On

Introduction

1 Helen Gould, *Miscarriage: An Enriching Experience*, unpublished MS.

Dreams and Dramas

1 Sheila Ernst and Lucy Goodison, *In Our Own Hands: A Book of Self-Help Therapy*, The Women's Press, 1981.
2 I first encountered this exercise in the form developed by Jan Dungey.
3 Peter Redgrove and Penelope Shuttle, *The Wise Wound: Menstruation and Everywoman*, Routledge and Kegan Paul, 1980.

Life Before Birth

1 A. J. Solter, *The Aware Baby: A New Approach to Parenting*, Shining Star Press, 1984.
2 T. Verny (with J. Kelly), *The Secret Life of the Unborn Child*, Sphere Books, 1982.
3 R. Ridgeway, *The Unborn Child: How to Recognise and Overcome Prenatal Trauma*, Wildwood House, 1987.
4 S. Kitzinger, *Being Born*, Dorling Kindersley, 1986.
5 A. Piontelli, *From Fetus to Child: An Observational and Psychoanalytic Study*, Routledge, 1992.
6 Ibid., p. 93.
7 Ibid., p. 98.
8 Ibid., p. 107.
9 J. Woodward, 'The Bereaved Twin', Proceedings of the International Congress of Twin Studies, 1986, Rome: AGMG.
10 Ibid., p. 6.
11 Piontelli, op. cit., p. 242.

2
Bibliography

The list of articles, pamphlets and books given below is by no means comprehensive but indicates those sources used most often in the preparation of *Hidden Loss*. In order to give the list some structure we have divided the books into sections but sometimes it has been difficult to decide how to categorise certain texts as their content crosses boundaries. We have marked some books in the Miscarriage section with an asterisk (*) to indicate those we would recommend from a feminist perspective or because they are written in a particularly sensitive and caring way.

Miscarriage and Other Pregnancy Loss

Berezin, N., *After a Loss in Pregnancy*, Fireside, New York, 1982.
* Borg, S. and Lasker, J., *When Pregnancy Fails*, Routledge and Kegan Paul, London, 1983.
Cooke, J., *Why Us Lord? The Trauma of Infertility: Personal Experiences*, Marshall Pickering, Basingstoke, 1985. Written from a Christian perspective.
de Gier, J., 'Miscarriage and Myths', *New Society*, 13 March 1987.
Fallaci, O., *Letter to a Child Never Born*, Hamalyn, London, 1976.
* Friedman, R. and Gradstein, B., *Surviving Pregnancy Loss*, Little, Brown & Company, New York, 1982. Distributed by Hutchinson Books.
Huisjes, H.J., *Spontaneous Abortion*, Churchill Livingstone, Edinburgh, 1984.
* Kane, R., *The Cervical Stitch: What it's Like*, The Miscarriage Association, 1986.
Lachelin, G. C. L., *Miscarriage: The Facts*, Oxford University Press, Oxford, 1985.
* Leroy, M., *Miscarriage*, Optima, in co-operation with The Miscarriage Association, London, 1988.
Lovell, A., 'When a baby dies', *New Society*, 4 August 1983, p. 167.
Maitland, S., 'Blessed are those who mourn', in *Telling Tales*, Journeyman Press, London, 1983. A story about miscarriage.

* National Childbirth Trust, *Miscarriage*. Available from local branches or Alexandra House, Oldham Terrace, London W3 6NH.
* Oakley, A., McPherson, A. and Roberts, H., *Miscarriage*, Fontana, London, 1984.
* Pfeiffer, N. and Woollett, A., *The Experience of Infertility*, Virago, London, 1983. Chapter 8 is on miscarriage.
Pfeiffer, N. and Woollett, A., *Women's Health and Infertility*, Women's Health Information Centre, London, 1986.
Pizer, H. and Palinski, C. O'Brien, *Coping with Miscarriage*, Jill Norman, London, 1980.
Pope, C., 'Miscarriage', *Peace News*, 20 February 1976, pp. 12–13.
Roberts, H., *Women's Health and Miscarriage*, Women's Health Information Centre, London, 1986.
Wilson, M., an account of miscarriage in S. Dowrick and S. Grundberg (eds.), *Why Children?*, The Women's Press, London, 1980.

Women, Maternity and Health

Barlow, S.M. and Sullivan, F.M., *Reproductive Hazards of Industrial Chemicals*, Academic Press, London, 1982.
Doyle, L., *The Political Economy of Health*, Pluto, London, 1979.
English, D. and Ehrenreich, B., *Complaints and Disorders: The Sexual Politics of Sickness*, Feminist Press, New York, 1973.
Fraser, J. L., *A Guide to Natural Medicine*, Thames/Methuen, London, 1981. An outline of natural therapies.
General Municipal Boilermakers and Allied Trades Union, *Your Reproductive Health at Risk*. Available from GMBATU, Thorne House, Ruxley Ridge, Claygate, Esher, Surrey KT10 OTL.
Gordon, L., *Woman's Body, Woman's Right: Birth Control in America*, Penguin, Harmondsworth, 1977.
Kitzinger, S., *The New Good Birth Guide*, Penguin, Harmondsworth, 1983.
Maternity Alliance, *Pregnant at Work, Getting Fit for Pregnancy* and *A Bibliography on Health before Pregnancy*. Leaflets available from 15 Britannia Street, London WC1X 9JP.
National Children's Bureau, 'Preconceptual and Early Antenatal Care: A Review of Research', *Highlight* No. 60. Leaflet available from 8 Wakley Street, London EC1V 7QE.

Neustatter, A. and Newson, G., *Mixed Feelings: The Experience of Abortion*, Pluto, London, 1986.

Nissim, R., *Natural Healing in Gynaecology: A Manual for Women*, Pandora, London, 1986.

Oakley, A., *Women Confined: Towards a Sociology of Chilbirth*, Martin Robertson, Oxford, 1980.

Parvati, J., *Hygeia: A Woman's Herbal*, Wildwood House, London, 1979.

Phillips, A., *Your Body, Your Baby, Your Life*, Pandora, London, 1983.

Phillips, A. and Rakusen, J. (eds.) *Our Bodies, Ourselves*, Penguin, Harmondsworth, 1987, revised 2nd edition.

Pickard, B., *Are You Fit Enough to Become Pregnant?, Be Fit and Healthy Before You Start a Baby*, 1983. Available from Lane End Farm, Denton, Ilkley, West Yorkshire LS29 OHP.

Pipes, M., *Understanding Abortion*, The Women's Press, London, 1986.

Rakusen, J. and Davidson, N., *Out of Our Hands: What Technology Does to Pregnancy*, Pan Books, London, 1982.

Redgrove, P. and Shuttle, P., *The Wise Wound: Menstruation and Everywoman*, Grafton, London, 1986, revised 2nd edition.

Turner, J. and Savage, W., *The Good Health Guide for Women*, Hamyln, London, 1981.

Weideger, P., *Female Cycles*, The Women's Press, London, 1978.

Wynn, M. and Wynn, A., *Lead and Human Reproduction*, 1982. Available from the CLEAR Charitable Trust, 2 Northdown Street, London N1 9BG.

Femininity and the Social Construction of Gender

Brownmiller, S., *Femininity*, Hamish Hamilton, London, 1984.

Chodorow, N., *The Reproduction of Mothering*, University of California Press, Los Angeles, 1978.

de Beauvoir, S., *The Second Sex*, Penguin, Harmondsworth, 1972.

Griffin, C, *Typical Girls*, Routledge and Kegan Paul, London, 1985.

Lees, S., *Losing Out: Sexuality and Adolescent Girls*, Hutchinson, London, 1986.

New, C. and David, M., *For the Children's Sake: Making Children More than Women's Business*, Penguin, Harmondsworth, 1985.

O'Brien, M., *The Politics of Reproduction*, Routledge and Kegan Paul, London, 1983.

Rich, A., *Of Woman Born: Motherhood as Experience and Institution*, Virago, London, 1979.

Rowbotham, S., *Woman's Consciousness, Man's World*, Penguin, Harmondsworth, 1973.

Parenting from Conception Onwards

Arcana, J., *Our Mother's Daughters*, The Women's Press, London, 1981.

— *Every Mother's Son*, The Women's Press, London, 1983.

Flanagan, G. L., *The First Nine Months of Life*, Pocket Books, New York, 1966. From conception to birth.

Itzin, C., 'Counselling on Prebirth Experiences', *Present Time*, No. 58, January 1985, pp. 27–8.

— 'Getting our Prebirth Lives Out of Occlusion', *Present Time*, No. 62, January 1986, pp. 35–6.

Kitzinger, S., with photographs by Nilsson, L., *Being Born*, Dorling Kindersley, London, 1986.

Miller, A., *Thou Shalt Not be Aware: Society's Betrayal of the Child*, Pluto, London, 1985.

— *The Drama of Being a Child*, Virago, London, 1987.

— *For Your Own Good: The Roots of Violence in Childrearing*, Virago, London, 1987.

Payne, K., *Between Ourselves: Letters Between Mothers and Daughters*, Picador, London, 1983.

Pearce, J. C., *Magical Child*, Bantam Books, London, 1986.

Solterm, A.J., *The Aware Baby: A New Approach to Parenting*, Shining Star Press, California, 1984.

Verny, T. and Kelly, J., *The Secret Life of the Unborn Child*, Sphere, London, 1982. Gives good medical and scientific information, but not a feminist point of view.

Therapy and Self-Help

Assaglioli, R., *Psychosynthesis*, Turnstone Press, Northamptonshire, 1986.

Dickson, A., *A Woman In Your Own Right: Assertiveness and You*, Quartet Books, London, 1982.

Eichenbaum, L. and Orbach, S., *Outside In Inside Out: Women's Psychology, a Feminist Psychoanalytic Approach*, Penguin, Harmondsworth, 1982.

— *What Do Women Want?* Fontana, London, 1981.

Ernst, S. and Goodison, L., *In Our Own Hands: A Book of Self-Help Therapy*, The Women's Press, London, 1981.

Faraday, A., *Dream Power*, Berkeley Books, New York, 1980.

Ferrucci, P., *What We May Be: The Visions and Techniques of Psychosynthesis*, Turnstone Press, Northamptonshire, 1986.

Itzin, C., 'Young People, Prebirth Distress and Pseudo-Survival Patterns', *Present Time*, No. 64, July 1986, pp. 60–2.

Jackins, T., 'Using co-counselling with the very young', in *The Caring Parent*, No. 3, 1983, pp. 3–4, Rational Island Publishers, Seattle.

Mariechild, D., *Mother Wit: Exercises for Healing, Growth and Spiritual Awareness*, Crossing Press, Freedom, California, 1981.

Murgatroyd, S. and Woolfe, R., *Coping with Crisis: Understanding and Helping People in Need*, Harper & Row, London, 1982.

Nairne, K. and Smith, G., *Dealing with Depression*, The Women's Press, London, 1983.

Parkes, C.M., *Bereavement: Studies of Grief in Adult Life*, Penguin: Harmondsworth, 1983 edn.

Perera, S. B., *Descent to the Goddess: A Way of Initiation for Women*, Inner City Books, 1981.

Rush, A.K., *Getting Clear, Bodywork for Women*, Wildwood House, London, 1974.

3
Glossary

Afterbirth

The afterbirth or placenta is the disc of specialised tissue that creates an interface between the foetal circulation and the mother's circulation within the womb. The foetus is connected to the afterbirth by the umbilical cord. It is across this disc of tissue that the foetus receives nutrition and oxygen from the mother's circulation, and then gets rid of waste products to the mother's circulation.

Alpha Feto Protein

This is a protein that can be measured in a blood sample taken from the mother as a screening procedure. If the level is raised this may indicate an increased risk of a spinal deformity in the foetus. If the level is low it may indicate a risk of Down's Syndrome. This protein is no longer measured in isolation but as part of the triple test.

Anti-D

An injection given to a rhesus negative woman after a miscarriage, ectopic pregnancy, termination of pregnancy or childbirth itself, to reduce the risk of rhesus problems in future pregnancies.

Azithromycin

A new antibiotic that is related to Erythromycin and has been introduced as a one dose treatment for chlamydia. There have been no studies to show whether it is safe during pregnancy or not.

Blighted ovum

A pregnancy where chromosomal abnormalities may lead to the formation of the placenta and membranes without an embryo; also referred to as an 'an embryonic' pregnancy.

Bromocriptine

A drug given in tablet form that acts to prevent the body's release of prolactin from the pituitary gland. As prolactin is important in breastfeeding, taking bromocriptine can make the milk dry up. It is offered to women as a two-week course after a late miscarriage or a stillbirth. It should be taken with food and can cause nausea and dizziness. After the course is stopped there may be some rebound milk production and often women prefer to avoid drugs at such a time and use simple pain-killers and a good supporting bra.

Cervix

The neck of the womb.

Dilatation and Curettage (D and C)

An operation where the cervix is dilated open and the lining of the womb scraped clean.

Down's Syndrome

Down's syndrome is a chromosomal problem where there are 47 chromosomes instead of the usual 46. The extra chromosome exists because there are three strands of chromosome 21 instead of two. Down's syndrome is therefore an example of 'trisomy'. There are other types of trisomy but they are usually incompatible with life, unlike Down's syndrome. The adult or child with Down's syndrome has characteristic facial features and learning disabilities. Common health problems are heart disease and diabetes.

Ectopic pregnancy

An ectopic pregnancy is one that starts to grow outside the uterus, usually in the fallopian tube. Characteristic symptoms are severe pain on one side of the abdomen, feelings of faintness and sometimes some bleeding from the vagina, usually by the tenth week of pregnancy. When an ectopic pregnancy is diagnosed, an operation to remove the pregnancy and tube is necessary, as the tube may burst leading to internal bleeding.

Epidural

A technique used to relieve pain during a late spontaneous or induced abortion, during labour or sometimes after abdominal surgery. An anaesthetist inserts a fine plastic catheter (epidural catheter) into the epidural space in the lower back. The epidural space is the space surrounding the spinal cord through which the emerging nerves pass before leaving the bony protection of the vertebrae. Local anaesthetic or pain-killing drugs can be injected at intervals through the catheter to provide the woman with pain relief. The local anaesthetic is the usual drug used to take away the pains of contractions. This drug is also likely to make the woman's legs feel numb. The pain-killing drugs are used to relieve pain after surgery and do not create numbness. When the drugs are no longer required the fine plastic catheter is removed.

Ergometrine

A powerful drug which makes the uterus contract and therefore helps stop heavy bleeding either during an early miscarriage or after the placenta is delivered in a late miscarriage. As its main side effect is severe vomiting it is less commonly given and Syntometrine or Syntocinon is preferred.

Erythromycin

A broad spectrum antibiotic that also has activity against chlamydia and is safe to use in pregnancy. It is also used for the treatment of ureaplasma and mycoplasma infections.

Evacuation of Retained Products of Conception (ERPC)

An operation performed to empty the womb under general anaesthetic, when a miscarriage is inevitable or incomplete in the first trimester.

Hydatidiform mole

A chromosomal problem, occurring in about one in 2,000 pregnancies in the UK. The mole is made up of an abnormal placenta consisting of thousands of small grape-like blobs. The embryo is rarely present, but can be. The woman may feel sick because the mole produces high levels of pregnancy hormones (HCG). The uterus appears to be bigger than her dates, and she may have noticed bleeding from the vagina, or even seen one of the grape-like blobs pass out.

Hysterosalpingogram (HSG)

A special X-ray to check the shape of the cavity of the uterus, and patency of the tubes.

Intra-uterine contraceptive device (IUCD)

More commonly known as the coil.

Laparoscopy

A telescope is inserted through a cut in the umbilicus under general anaesthesia. After this some carbon dioxide gas is introduced through a fine needle inserted through the same cut. A small cut may also be necessary either just above the pubic hairline or to the left or right side. This is to introduce another instrument that can help move the fallopian tubes and ovaries about in order to get a better view. If the entire operation is performed with a laparoscope there will be at least two of these extra cuts which will only be 1–2cm in length and should heal with the minimum of scarring.

Laparotomy

This is the operation to enter the abdomen and pelvis which is necessary if there has been major haemorrhage from a ruptured ectopic pregnancy or if a salpingectomy is necessary. It may also be necessary if the salpingostomy or milking out of an ectopic pregnancy cannot be performed through the laparoscope. Usually this incision is small, about 3–4 inches long, and is made either just above or just in the top of the pubic hairline. Often it is closed with a dissolvable stitch.

Methotrexate

A drug commonly used in chemotherapy for leukaemia. It kills cells by interfering with their folate mechanism which is essential for cell replication. Methotrexate can be used in the medical treatment of a small unruptured ectopic pregnancy that is not bleeding and shows no foetal heart activity on scan. Methotrexate has been used as a direct injection into the foetal sac in the tube using transvaginal ultrasound to guide the injection. Alternatively it is given to the woman via an injection into the vein or muscle as a course of treatment over several days.

Miscarriage

The medical terms used to describe a miscarriage need some explanation. Usually the medical profession refers to a miscarriage as an abortion, as discussed on pp. 55–6.

Threatened miscarriage (abortion)

This term is used when there has been some bleeding and perhaps a little pain, but the neck of the womb remains closed and an ultrasound scan confirms that the pregnancy is still continuing.

Inevitable miscarriage (abortion)

A miscarriage becomes inevitable once the neck of the womb begins to open. This is normally accompanied by more pain and bleeding. After 12 weeks of pregnancy another sign of an inevitable miscarriage would be an awareness of the waters coming away. Sometimes the waters break when the baby is quite big and close to the time when it might survive. In this situation a miscarriage is not always inevitable. The water around the baby is continually being reformed, and providing there is no infection present, the pregnancy can continue; however, once the neck of the womb begins to open, the miscarriage does become inevitable.

Incomplete miscarriage (abortion)

This is the next stage and is usually accompanied by more pain and bleeding. The term incomplete means that the womb has passed some of the pregnancy tissue but not all of it has come away. The further advanced the pregnancy, the more frightening and painful this stage can be, especially if a recognisable baby is passed. The womb tends to continue to bleed until it is empty and thus to hasten this process, and to stop the bleeding and any risk of infection, it is usual for doctors to perform an operation to empty the womb completely. This operation is referred to as an Evacuation of Retained Products of Conception (ERPC).

Complete miscarriage (abortion)

Sometimes the womb empties itself completely and an operation is not necessary.

Septic miscarriage (abortion)

If a miscarriage is incomplete and the remaining tissue is not removed, this tissue can form a focus for infection. Infection is fortunately not common these days. Before the 1967 Abortion Act it was seen in women who had illegal terminations of pregnancy.

A missed abortion

This is a difficult situation to understand. What happens is that the pregnancy comes to an end but the womb does not empty straight away. It can be several months before this happens spontaneously. The woman may suspect a problem because she no longer feels pregnant. The womb will feel smaller than expected for the time from the last period and the neck of the womb will be closed. An ultrasound scan will confirm suspicions. This situation is frequently associated with an anembryonic pregnancy (see *Blighted Ovum*, above), and occurs in the first trimester. Sometimes it occurs in the second trimester following the death of the baby, perhaps because of abnormalities. The longer the baby and pregnancy tissue remain inside the womb, the greater the risk of disturbance to the woman's blood-clotting mechanisms. Thus when this problem is discovered it is important to empty the womb and to check the woman's blood for any clotting problems.

Elective abortion, therapeutic abortion and termination of pregnancy

These are the terms used when a woman decides to end her pregnancy and the baby and other contents of the uterus are removed. At the time of writing, a pregnancy may be terminated up to 24 weeks, for social and medical reasons, with the signatures of two doctors. The baby may be removed using vacuum aspiration (the preferred method for pregnancies up to 16 weeks), by dilatation of the cervix and evacuation (a D and E) of the uterine contents, or by the use of prostaglandins to induce labour for pregnancies over 16 weeks.

Pethidine

A synthetic drug related to morphine. It acts as a powerful painkiller and may be given for the pain of a miscarriage or an ectopic pregnancy or after any operation. It is usually given into the muscle of the thigh or buttock and often combined with another drug to stop the feeling of sickness.

Polyploidy

Polyploidy is an extreme form of chromosomal abnormality and is the name given to chromosomal complements occurring in excess of the normal 46 chromosomes (23 pairs). Polyploidy occurs in multiples of 23, e.g.: triploidy refers to 69 pairs; tetraploidy, to 92; and so on. Polyploidy is found in anembryonic pregnancies and hydatidiform moles.

Salpingectomy

Removal of all or part of the fallopian tube. Still the standard surgery for a ruptured ectopic pregnancy or an ectopic pregnancy in the tube already damaged by previous infection or surgery.

Salpingostomy

The fallopian tube is cut open over the site of the ectopic pregnancy. Pregnancy tissue is removed and any bleeding controlled. The incision may be left open to heal or may be closed with very fine sutures.

Syntocinon

A synthetic form of the body's natural hormone oxytocin. Syntocinon acts to contract the uterus and stop bleeding. It can be given by injection into the muscle or diluted in fluid in an intravenous drip. It is often given intraveneously during an ERPC.

Syntometrine

A mixture of syntocinon and ergometrine given as an injection into the muscle to contract the uterus and stop bleeding. Usually given after the delivery of the placenta in the late miscarriage or delivery of a baby at term.

Tetracyclines

A group of antibiotics that have a specific action against chlamydia. They should not be given during pregnancy as they can discolour the developing teeth of the baby.

Trimester

Pregnancy is divided into three parts, known as trimesters. The first trimester is from conception up to 14 weeks; the second is between 14 and 24 weeks; and the third is from 24 weeks until delivery.

Turner's Syndrome

This is a chromosomal abnormality that can be compatible with life, but is also found in a proportion of aborted foetuses. The chromosomal problem arises because there are only 45 chromosomes instead of the usual 46. The missing chromosome is one of the X sex chromosomes. An adult with Turner's syndrome will appear to be female, is usually short and is often diagnosed at puberty because her periods do not start. The diagnosis may be made earlier because of typical features such as webbing of the neck. A woman with Turner's syndrome is not fertile.

Ultrasound scan

A scan which helps the doctor to see whether the developing baby appears to be normal, it cannot show up all foetal abnormalities but will help to detect major physical abnormalities that could be life threatening.

4
What Happens During the First Nine Months of Life

The First Month

Week One. The embryo begins to take shape from the group of cells in the wall of the womb.

Week Two. An embryonic shield containing the preliminary tissues for all of the body is formed.

Week Three. The embryonic shield has developed into an amnion enclosing a beating heart, brain, spinal cord and precursors for vertebrae; the whole structure is 1.5 mm long.

Week Four. A whole embryo is now formed. It has a body, a head, the beginnings of eyes, a mouth and ears, a beating heart and blood stream, and a brain showing human specialisation. In this week arm buds appear.

The Second Month

Week Five. The arms, hands, and shoulders are forming and then finger outlines begin to show on the hands. Pigment forms in the retina of the eyes.

Week Six. There is a complete skeleton of cartilage.

Week Seven. The embryo is 18 mm long, and has all the internal organs and features of the future adult. It weighs $\frac{1}{30}$ ounce. It has a human face, with all the features, and the beginnings of milk teeth are in its gums. The foetus has muscles and is covered by a thin skin. Arms have hands with fingers and thumbs. Legs have knees, ankles and toes. The heart is beating and the brain, kidneys and stomach are all actively functioning. The liver is making blood cells.

Week Eight. The cartilage skeleton is replaced by bone cells. The soles of the feet and the palms of the hands are already permanently lined.

The Third Month

Weeks Nine and Ten. Nerve/muscle connections increase three-fold, nail beds are forming on fingertips. The eyelids close and will remain shut until the sixth month. Ribs and vertebrae turn to hard bone.

By Week 12 the foetus can kick, turn her feet and curl her toes, can grimace and squint, and open her mouth, and swallow. Lips form and the sucking muscles fill out in the cheeks, while taste buds and saliva glands appear. External genitalia have formed in both sexes from virtually identical folds of tissue. Internal reproductive organs form. The foetus has working digestive glands in the stomach and sometimes urinates.

The Fourth Month

In this month the foetus grows to 20–25 cm in length and weighs 6 ounces. It is during the fourth month that the placenta, which provides the foetus with food, oxygen and water, is properly formed.

The Fifth Month

The foetus grows to 30 cm in length, weighs one pound, and has hair, eyebrows and lashes. The skeleton hardens and hard nails form on fingers and toes. The heartbeat is louder. The baby has hiccups. A distinct pattern of sleeping and waking emerges.

The Sixth Month

By this month the baby is about 35 cm long, with a little fat under the skin. She weighs ¼ pounds. Permanent teeth buds appear, and the baby's eyelids can open and she may look up, down and to the side. She develops a strong grip, and can suck, make a fist, kick, punch and somersault. If born prematurely during the sixth month, the baby is capable of maintaining regular breathing and can survive in an incubator although the lungs and digestive system are usually too immature to take over their full functions.

Months Seven, Eight and Nine

It is now that the baby gains most of her birthweight, putting on more than a pound in the seventh month and probably four more in the following six weeks. Research has shown that the foetus can hear and respond to sound; is responsive to pressure and touch; sucks, drinks and swallows, responding to sweet and bitter tastes; hiccups and responds to pain.

5
Resources

Miscarriage and Other Pregnancy Loss

ISSUE (National Fertility Association)
509 Aldridge Road
Great Barr
Birmingham B44 8NA
Telephone 0121 344 4414
Publishes fact sheets on infertility and miscarriage.

The Miscarriage Association
c/o Clayton Hospital
Northgate
Wakefield
West Yorkshire WF1 3JS
Telephone 01924 200799
Offers information and support for women who have had mis-
carriages. Publishes a newsletter, a booklet on the cervical stitch,
and runs self-help groups throughout the country.

National Childbirth Trust
Alexandra House
Oldham Terrace
London W3 6NH
Telephone 0181 992 8637
Runs support groups around the country.

SAFTA (Support Around Termination for Foetal Abnormality)
73 Charlotte Street
London W1P 1LB
Telephone 0171 631 0280 (Admin)
            0171 631 0285 (Helpline)

SANDS (The Stillbirth and Neonatal Death Society)
28 Portland Place
London W1N 3DE
Telephone 0171 436 5881 (Helpline)
            0171 436 7940 (Information)

TAMBA (The Twins and Multiple Births Association)
PO Box 30
Little Sutton
South Wirral L66 1TH
Telephone 0151 348 0020
Offers support where one twin (or member of multiple birth set)
dies and is miscarried. Publishes a newsletter and leaflets.

Tommy's Campaign
7th Floor
North Wing
St Thomas' Hospital
London SE1 7EH
National charity funding research into prematurity, miscarriage
and stillbirth.

Women's Information Centres

Women's Health (WH)
52–4 Featherstone Street
London EC1
Telephone 0171 251 6580
Provides information on most aspects of women's health and
reproduction and a range of broadsheets on specific areas,
including miscarriage. Also has a reference library.

Pregnancy and Health Care

Association for Improvements in the Maternity Services (AIMS)
c/o 40 Kingswood Avenue
London NW6 6LS
Telephone 0181 960 5585
Offers sympathetic advice on parents' rights in all aspects of
maternity care. Helpline Monday–Friday, 9am–6pm.

British Diabetic Association
10 Queen Anne Street
London W1M OBD
Telephone 0171 323 1531

Endometriosis Association
Suite 50
Westminster Palace Gardens
1–7 Artillery Row
London SW1P 1RL
Telephone 0171 222 2776
Crisis support line 7–10pm

Foresight
(The Association for the Promotion of Pre-Conceptual Care)
28 The Paddock
Goldaming
Surrey GU7 1XD
Telephone 01483 427839
Provides a wide range of booklets and information on pre-
conception care, with particular provision for post-miscarriage
couples.

Health and Safety Executive
Rose Court
2 Southwark Bridge
London SE1 9HS
Telephone 0171 717 6000
Responsible for enforcing the law which limits exposure to hazards
at work.

The Health Education Authority
Hamilton House
Mabledon Place
London WC1H 9TX
Telephone 0171 383 3833

The Maternity Alliance
15 Britannia Street
London WC1X 9JP
Telephone 0171 837 1265
Publishes leaflets free to individuals, on receipt of sae.

Sickle Cell Society
54 Station Road
London NW10 4UA
Telephone 0181 961 7795

City Centre
32–5 Featherstone Street
London EC1Y 8QX
Telephone 0171 608 1338 (Helpline)
Provides literature and advice for office workers on VDU health and safety, etc.

Therapies

Assertiveness Training. Local education authorities sometimes offer courses, or write to Anne Dickson (author of *A Woman In Your Own Right*), c/o Quartet Books Ltd, 27–9 Goodge Street, London W1P 1FD

Women's Therapy Centre
6–9 Manor Gardens
London N7
Telephone 0171 263 6200

Alternative Medicine

The Acupuncture Association and Register
34 Alderney Street
London SW1V 4EU
London 0171 834 1012

British Homeopathic Association
27a Devonshire Street
London W1N 1RJ
Telephone 0171 935 2163
Publishes booklet on homeopathy for midwives and pregnant women.

The General Council and Register of Naturopaths
Frazer House
6 Netherhall Gardens
London NW3 5RR
Telephone 0171 435 8728
         01458 840072 (Helpline)

National Institute of Medical Herbalists
56 Longbrook Street
Exeter
Devon EX4 6AH
Telephone 01392 426022

School of Phytotherapy (Herbal Medicine)
Bucksteep Manor
Bodle Street Green
Nr Hailsham
East Sussex BN27 4RJ
Telephone 01323 833812/4

6
Notes on Contributors

Kirsten Duckitt is a Registrar in Obstetrics and Gynaecology at Addenbrookes Hospital, Cambridge.

Marilyn Duker was, at the time of writing, a mother, therapist and writer. She co-authored *Anorexia Nervosa and Bulimia: How to Help* (Open University Press, 1988) with her husband Roger Slade. As a therapist, she works with both women and men, in groups and individually.

Janet Grant was, at the time of writing, an educational psychologist with a university career in the field of health and social welfare. She has worked for the World Health Organisation Task Force on Human Reproduction, developing educational programmes on natural family planning.

Penny Henrion has written poetry and a play. She performed with the Bloody Poets for a time and co-founded a lesbian theatre group, MOWTH. She has worked in education and community development, and now manages a small charity which supports carers. She lives in Reading, and is delighted to be a mother to Luke and Julia.

Lindsay James is a pseudonym. She is a mother, a therapist and a counsellor working in private practice with women and men.

Carla Shagass Kelley was, at the time of writing, an attorney practising employment law in Portland, Oregon, USA.

Helen McNeil is a writer and a teacher. She is married to the sculptor Graham Ashton and has two children, Liberty and Gabriel. Helen divides her time between London and Norwich, where she lectures in American literature, women's studies and film studies at the University of East Anglia. Her critical study *Emily Dickinson* was published by Virago in 1986 and she is working on two novels and further critical books.

Fran Reader is Consultant in Family Planning and Reproductive

Health Care at Ipswich Hospital. She is a trained psycho-sexual counsellor and has counselled many women over the range of issues around reproduction, including abortion counselling, termination of abnormality and preconceptual counselling. Fran has two children, Philip and Emily.

Phil Scraton was, at the time of writing, a Principal Lecturer in Criminology at Edge Hill College of Higher Education, Ormskirk.

Sheila Scraton was, at the time of writing, a lecturer at Leeds Polytechnic living with Phil, Paul and Sean in Lancashire.

Ann Wickham has three children, two boys and a girl. At the time of writing, she worked in distance education in Ireland.

Gill Yudkin is a GP in a group practice in North London with a particular interest in women's health issues. She has two grown-up children, Harriet and Josh. Gill was a founder member of the Women's Health Information Centre (now Women's Health).

Index